Manual of
GI Fluoroscopy

Manual of GI Fluoroscopy

Bruce R. Javors M.D.

Professor of Clinical Radiology,
University of Medicine and Dentistry–
New Jersey Medical School
Chief, Diagnostic Radiology
V.A. Medical Center, East Orange, NJ

Illustrations by
Sue Cohen

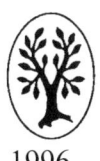

SOUTH UNIVERSITY
709 MALL BLVD.
SAVANNAH, GA 31406

1996

Thieme Medical Publishers, Inc., New York
Georg Thieme Verlag, Stuttgart • *New York*

Thieme Medical Publishers, Inc.
381 Park Avenue South
New York, NY 10010

MANUAL OF GI FLUOROSCOPY
Bruce Javors

Library of Congress Cataloging-in-Publication Data

Copyright © 1996 by Thieme Medical Publishers, Inc. This book, including all parts thereof, is legally protected by copyright. Any use, exploitation or commercialization outside the narrow limits set by copyright legislation, without the publisher's consent, is illegal and liable to prosecution. This applies in particular to photostat reproduction, copying, mimeographing or duplication of any kind, translating, preparation of microfilms, and electronic data processing and storage.

Important Note: Medicine is an ever-changing science. Research and clinical experience are continually broadening our knowledge, in particular our knowledge of proper treatment and drug therapy. Insofar as this book mentions any dosage or application, readers may rest assured that the authors, editors, and publishers have made every effort to ensure that such references are strictly in accordance with the state of knowledge at the time of production of the book. Nevertheless, every user is requested to carefully examine the manufacturer's leaflets accompanying each drug to check on his own responsibility whether the dosage schedules recommended therein or the contraindications stated by the manufacturers differ from the statements made in the present book. Such examination is particularly important with drugs that are either rarely used or have been newly released on the market.

Some of the product names, patents, and registered designs referred to in this book are in fact registered trademarks or proprietary names even though specific reference to this fact is not always made in the text. Therefore, the appearance of a name without designation as proprietary is not to be construed as a representation by the publisher that it is in the public domain.

Printed in the United States of America

54321

TMP ISBN 0-86577-607-5
GTV ISBN 3-13-102681-2

Dedication

Dedicated to my parents, Sam and Sylvia, for instilling within me a love of both education and medicine, which I have been fortunate enough to combine in my career; and to my wife Sue and daughter Alli for having endured many lonely hours and lost days and weekends while I sat at the computer. Their love and affection have sustained me through this volume's long gestation and sometimes difficult delivery.

ACKNOWLEDGEMENTS

The author gratefully acknowledges the strong support of the E-Z-Em Corporation in providing an educational grant that underwrote large portions of this book's preparation. In particular, Howard Stern and Gloria Riina deserve special attention.

Over two decades ago, Emil Balthazar started me down the road of GI radiology and I am still happily pursuing that path. Hank Goldberg and the late Tom Beneventano provided me with guidance when I got lost amongst the thickets. Along the way I have had the great pleasure to personally study with and learn from Dean Maglinte and Professor the late Hikoo Shirakabee, amongst many others. As always, I am solely responsible for all they taught me and that I have forgotten or misquoted.

After almost 20 years of working alongside and teaching residents, I must acknowledge their inspiration and support for this project through its many stages. They have always been instrumental in asking me not only how to do things, but more importantly why.

My medical artist, Sue Cohen, also deserves special thanks. She has had the unenvious job of taking my rough, and sometimes almost indecipherable sketches and converting them into the wonderful illustrations that grace this book. Working against severe time pressure, she has performed beyond expectation.

Last, but not least, I must acknowledge the strong support of my editor, Jane Pennington, who saw this project through, from its rough beginnings to its finale.

Contents

Dedication *v*
Acknowledgements *vii*
Preface *xiii*

GENERAL PRINCIPLES 1

1 PHARYNX AND ESOPHAGUS—ROUTINE 21

Pharyngogram *23*
Rapid Sequence Cervical Esophagram *25*
Esophagus—Single Contrast *28*
Esophagus—Double Contrast *30*

2 PHARYNX AND ESOPHAGUS—SPECIAL 33

Esophageal Obstruction *35*
Esophageal Perforation *36*
Achalasia *38*
Esophageal Varices *40*
Retained Esophageal Foreign Body *41*
Tracheoesophageal Fistula *44*
Post-Esophagogastrectomy *46*
Post-Esophagojejunostomy *52*
Post-Colonic Interposition *56*
Celestine Tube Implant Study *58*

3 STOMACH—ROUTINE 61

Upper GI Series—Single Contrast *63*
Upper GI Series—Double Contrast *68*

4 STOMACH—SPECIAL 77

Salvaging the Failed Double Contrast Upper GI Series *79*
Posterior Duodenal Bulb Maneuver *83*
Outlet Obstruction *86*
Upper GI for Perforated Viscus *88*
Billroth II—Single Contrast *90*
Billroth II—Double Contrast *93*
Gastrostomy Tube *98*
Bypass Gastrojejunostomy Without Resection *100*
Gastrojejunostomy Without Resection—Double Contrast *104*
Gastric Stapling *109*

5 SMALL BOWEL—ROUTINE 111

Dedicated Small Bowel Study *113*
Enteroclysis Tube Placement *117*
Enteroclysis—Single Contrast *124*
Enteroclysis—Double Contrast *127*

6 SMALL BOWEL—SPECIAL 131

Peroral Pneumocolon *133*
Small Bowel Obstruction *135*
Small Bowel Perforation *137*
Ileostomy Study *139*
Ileoanal "J" or "S" Pouch *142*

7 COLON—ROUTINE 145

Single Contrast Barium Enema *147*
Double Contrast Barium Enema *151*
Dynamic Proctography (Defecography) *157*

CONTENTS

8 COLON—SPECIAL **161**

Salvaging the Failed Double Contrast Enema *163*
Colonic Obstruction *167*
Colonic Perforation *171*
End Colostomy *173*
Anterior Resection with Rectal Pouch (Hartmann Procedure) *176*
Double-Barrel Colostomy *181*
Rectovaginal Fistula *186*
Rectovesical Fistula *188*
Bourne Test *189*

9 PANCREAS/BILIARY TREE **191**

Endoscopic Retrograde Cholangiopancreatography (ERCP) *193*
T-tube Cholangiogram *197*
Nasobiliary Cholangiogram *202*
Oral Cholecystogram *205*
Cholecystostomy Tube Study *207*

10 MISCELLANEOUS **209**

Fistulogram *211*

APPENDICES **213**

I Patient Checklist *213*
II Sample Report *215*
III Patient Positioning Guide *219*

INDEX **229**

PREFACE

This book is designed for the neophyte fluoroscopist or those who have not been exposed to many of the newer techniques in gastrointestinal fluoroscopy. It would be presumptuous of me to think of these as the definitive ways to perform these procedures. However, they do represent the compilation of many different styles and techniques I have adapted over more than two decades of fluoroscoping and teaching.

If the reader wants to make any modifications or improvements in these instructions, then he or she should feel free to do so. Some of the techniques described are long and entail multiple position changes and many spot films. These reflect my principle interest in and practice of academic gastrointestinal radiology.

This book started as a compilation of various notes, drawings, and "cheat sheets" that were prepared as part of my teaching of GI fluoroscopy to incoming first-year radiology residents. Over the last decade the case load in fluoroscopy has decreased and, with this, so has the classic apprenticeship method of teaching. In most teaching departments this decrease in case load has been accompanied by a shift in interest of the attending radiologist in charge of GI to other imaging modalities. The result is that there has been even less personal oversight of the resident during fluoroscopy. More often than not, fluoroscopy is being taught by "junior attendings" or senior residents to more junior ones.

In order to bridge this gap in teaching, I have developed a systematic "cookbook" approach to instruct residents in the basics of fluoroscopy. Schematic drawings of the basic radiographic positions and line drawings representing the fluoroscopic image were added at the request of the residents. This was particularly advantageous when teaching one resident who was dyslexic and could not process the written instructions and envision them. Eventually I was approached by the E-Z-Em Corporation who, with an educational grant, supported expansion of my notes into a more comprehensive survey of GI procedures.

This volume of procedures is preceded by an introductory section that discusses the *General Principles* that underlie these techniques. Included are discussions of when to do single versus double contrast, when to use water soluble contrast, and how to handle frequently encountered, but potentially difficult situations.

The body of this text is comprised of the actual examinations, arranged by anatomic region. The core examinations are always discussed first within each region. These are then followed by variations of these exams necessitated by different clinical scenarios. Modifications are also discussed for other situations such as the post-operative setting. The discussion of each differing examination starts with suggestions regarding preliminary films and the type of contrast needed. Technologist-performed overheads are also enumerated. At the end of some examinations are *Notes* that further explain the examination and possible pitfalls.

The actual line-by-line instructions are accompanied by two types of illustrations. One, incorporated within the text, is a schematic of the patient position on the X-ray table. These are drawn as cross sections viewed from below, similar to CT scans. The second, and larger, figure is in the column opposite the text. This line drawing approximates how the fluoroscopic image should appear on the screen, and it has been drawn with the purpose of teaching proper positioning of the patient, rather than being a complete depiction of the anatomy and pathology that would be visualized in real life. The text always refers to the patient in the anatomic **(AP [SUPINE])** ⊕ position on the fluoroscopy table.

Appendix III includes line drawings that more fully depict the basic radiographic positions alongside the schematic diagrams. Appendix II is a *Sample Report* for an examination, with an analysis of the report and what should be contained within it; this reflects my personal bias, but it may be used as a foundation upon which a complete report is based. Another feature, in Appendix I, is a *Patient Checklist* of the pertinent questions that an examiner should ask of the patient before proceeding with a test. In addition, it contains places to write the schedule for delayed films and for the fluoroscopist to record his or her contemporaneous interpretation of the fluoroscopic findings.

Similar to ultrasound, fluoroscopy is very operator-dependent and requires knowledge of anatomy and physiology as well as considerable practice. However, "Painting with Barium" can be very rewarding, both to the patient and the successful practitioner of the art. I hope that the reader will find these instructions helpful and that their interest in GI radiology will be enhanced or refreshed.

Bruce R. Javors, M.D.

GENERAL PRINCIPLES

Selecting the Best Examination

The exam that best answers the clinical problem is the one that should be chosen. This can be decided by reviewing the appropriate clinical information: by reading the clinical information available on the requisition, reviewing the patient's chart, speaking to the ordering physician, and—sometimes most importantly (but least often done)—speaking to and examining the patient.

Further information should be obtained by reviewing other studies that the patient may have undergone. These may include CT, US, and MRI, as well as prior fluoroscopic and routine examinations.

A short checklist for pertinent historical information is included in Appendix I.

Scout Films

Although the cost–benefit analysis of preliminary films (especially for the evaluation of colon preparation prior to the performance of a barium enema) has been called into question, we still advocate use of the practice. It is unusual for significant retained stool to be present, but not detectable in our practice. The additional information gained (anatomic as well as pathologic) in our opinion certainly outweighs the added cost and radiation exposure.

In addition to preliminary films, preliminary fluoroscopic examination of the chest and abdomen may reveal significant information that was not apparent on the original film. This is especially true in fluoroscoping the heart, where vascular and valvular calcifications are exquisitely demonstrated in their dynamic state but extremely difficult to see on a static film.

When preliminary films are obtained, they should be anatomically appropriate to the study. For a UGI series and an ERCP, the superior edge of the film should include the domes of the diaphragm. For an SBS or BE, the inferior edge should include the area immediately below the pubic symphysis to the level of the obturator foramen. If two films are necessary for complete coverage from diaphragm to obturator foramen, then both should be obtained. For an OCG, a coned-down view of the RUQ should be obtained, in addition to a full abdominal film centered as for a UGI. For esophagrams, a well-penetrated Bucky film of the chest should precede the exam. For rapid sequence cervical esophagrams and pharyngograms films of the neck, soft tissue (low kVp) technique should be used.

Additional films should be obtained as warranted. These can include upright films of the chest or left lateral decubitus films of the abdomen to evaluate for free intraperitoneal air before examing a patient with an acute abdomen. In patients in whom it is difficult to differentiate a paralytic ileus from a low-lying colonic obstruction, a left lateral film of the pelvis (similar to the lateral rectal film from a single contrast BE) may allow air to rise from the descending and sigmoid colons to reach the rectum in the former but not the latter. This may obviate the need for a contrast exam. In utilizing all of these additional views, sufficient time must be allowed to permit free air to shift. Therefore, at least a five-minute interval should follow the change in position prior to filming.

If the preliminary film shows residual contrast from a prior exam (barium or CT), repeat the film at the higher kVp (100 to 135) at which the diagnostic examination would be performed. This will give a more accurate depiction of the opacity rendered by the retained contrast and, further, would allow a diagnostic study to be performed that might otherwise have been canceled.

Radiation Dose to the Examiner

First, any persons involved in radiology and, more importantly, fluoroscopy should be reconciled to the idea that their job entails exposing themselves to ionizing radiation. What should concern examiners is how to maximize the information obtained during fluoroscopy while minimizing their dosage of radiation. The best ways to minimize exposure are the following:

1. *Shorten the procedure time,* but not at the expense of the diagnostic quality of the examination. Paradoxically, this usually means turning the patient under direct fluoroscopic guidance. Although this seems to entail increased exposure time, it actually decreases it by eliminating the constant repositioning and subsequent reexposure caused by the resultant under and/or overrotation allowed when the patient is "blindly" turned.

2. *Remember the inverse square law.* Keep the fluoroscopy tower as close to the patient as possible at all times. This also gives you the added bonus of sharper images (secondary to decreased geometric unsharpness).

3. *Shield thyself.* Use a lead apron and thyroid shield at all times. Leaded eyeglasses (planar or prescription) are recommended for those who plan to continue fluoroscoping after residency. Leaded gloves should be worn if the hands approach the direct fluoroscopy beam. Lightweight leaded latex gloves are available for special procedures in which manual dexterity must be preserved. Remember, lead only works if it is between you and the X-ray source. If you turn sideways during a procedure, have a separate lead shield available (on a stand) or use a wraparound apron. Use all the appropriate shielding available on the fluoroscopy table (flaps that cover the Bucky tray access, moveable curtains on the fluoroscopy tower, etc.).

4. *Distance is another way of decreasing your exposure.* Obviously, a remote control room is the ultimate defense. Otherwise,

operating the fluoroscopy unit at arm's length offers some small degree of additional protection.
5. *Compression paddles* and spoonlike devices allow examiners to compress loops of bowel or lesions, or determine the mobility of various structures, without placing their hands in the direct beam.

Single Contrast Examinations

Single contrast or solid column studies depend on the visualization of abnormal indentations of masses into or projections of contrast outside the normal lumen. These are usually best seen in profile, and therefore, multiple obliquities are needed to see as much, if not all, of the circumference of the bowel in profile. In addition, "en face" visualization of lesions is possible and very often needed.

In order to obtain this information, the solid column of barium must be adequately penetrated by the X-ray beam. Three major factors affect this penetration. One is the kVp of the primary X-ray beam. Obviously, the higher the kVp, the more penetrating the beam is. The inherent loss of contrast from using a high kVp is more than offset by the high contrast of the barium–soft tissue interface.

The second factor is the density of the barium suspension used. In the larger diameter colon, a very low-density barium (15 to 20 percent w/v) is needed to allow adequate penetration, especially in areas of overlapping loops of bowel. In the stomach and small intestine, a higher density (35 to 50 percent w/v) is used. In addition, this higher density usually allows sufficiently dense coating of the mucosa to permit limited air contrast views of the stomach and duodenal bulb. In the esophagus, when it is examined by itself—and not as part of an upper GI series—an even higher-density barium (70 to 80 percent w/v) may be used.

The third factor is compression. In order to penetrate the solid column of barium, external compression (by a device attached to the fluoroscopy unit, a cone on a manual handle, or a balloon paddle) decreases the A-P diameter of the bowel examined. In addition, the compression allows the examiner to evaluate the distensibility of the bowel as well as its mobility. Fine detail of the surface characteristics, as well as the nature of the base or attachment of a filling defect, are seen to better advantage with compression. Overlying loops of bowel may sometimes be moved away from the area of interest, especially when the compression is applied in an oblique manner (not possible with the usual units attached to the fluoroscopy tower). In the colon the use of vigorous compression allows the examiner to move and occassionally fragment fecal material into smaller particles, thereby allowing better visualization of small polypoid lesions. It should be noted that areas such as the gastric fundus, splenic flexure, and the distal rectosigmoid colon are difficult to compress, due to the overlying rib cage and pelvic bones respectively.

Double Contrast Studies

The techniques and materials used for double contrast studies differ markedly from those used in single contrast. Visualization of raised or ulcerated lesions depends on adequate coating of the mucosa by dense barium, along with distention provided by air (in the esophagus, stomach, and colon) or methylcellulose (in the small bowel).

It is not always necessary to see lesions both in profile and "en face." Instead, it is often desirable to see the lesion on both the dependent surface (partially covered by the barium pool) *and* on the nondependent surface (coated only by barium and surrounded by air); thus, the oblique films obtained in single contrast studies are not as critical in double contrast examinations. In addition, the use of obliques to "open up" the flexures (or to see through two otherwise overlapping loops of bowel) is not as important because it is much easier to see through two air-filled loops. However, careful attention to the use of oblique positioning is necessary to deliver the barium to allow adequate coating of the mucosal surface. This requires strict attention to detail and the exact sequence of coating and air-filling of the bowel.

In the stomach and esophagus, the barium used must be of sufficiently high density to allow excellent visualization of mucosal detail with a microscopically thin layer coating the mucosa. Yet, the barium must be of low enough viscosity that it flows readily and can penetrate the small gastric grooves (area gastricae) as well as other mucosal markings. In Japan, barium of 150 to 160 percent w/v is used; in the United States, the barium is usually approximately 250 percent w/v. In the colon, a density of 100 percent w/v is sufficient. For the small bowel enema, a barium of 70 to 80 percent w/v is needed. All of these special double contrast bariums contain special additives that prevent the formation of bubbles and promote adherence to the mucosal surface, as well as governing its flow characteristics and storage potential. Antifungal and antibacterial agents are also added to maintain product safety.

Double contrast agents used differ by the organ examined. For the esophagus and stomach, a coarse powder or granules containing mainly sodium bicarbonate is used. An acidifying agent is also part of the formula. When dissolved in water, carbon dioxide is liberated. This must be formulated so that it does not dissolve too rapidly in the mouth because the gas will not then enter the GI tract; or too slowly so that the stomach is not properly distended because it will then be filled with undissolved granules. In addition, antifoaming agents are added to prevent bubble formation. In the colon, gas is introduced manually through a separate channel in the enema tip. Room air is usually used, although there are some theoretical as well as practical advantages to using carbon dioxide. These include the much more rapid absorption of the distending gas, decreasing the duration of the discomfort caused by the marked colonic distention. No cases of hypercarbia have been reported. The cumbersome nature, safety issues, and cost of carbon dioxide delivery systems have limited their adaptation in most centers. In the small bowel, a 0.5 percent aqueous methyl cellulose solution is used routinely as the double contrast agent. The methylcellulose propels the barium forward, distends the lumen, and prevents diffusion of the barium into the aqueous component (thereby avoiding the dilution of the barium). The Japanese are fond of using air as the distending agent; however, air tends to rise to the top of the small bowel loops causing distention and cramps, rather than propelling the barium in an antegrade manner. The Japanese report sucessful double contrast of the terminal ileum in only 60 to 70 percent of patients.

Fluoroscopy Units

Although any modern fluoroscopy unit uses image intensification and therefore administers a sufficiently low dose to both examiner and patient, there are certain components and features that can enhance its capabilities and usefulness:

1. A *multiformat spot film device* that allows large format (25×30 or 35×35 cm) cassettes to be used. These large cassettes allow such wide anatomic coverage that they can replace the technologist-performed "overhead" films in many examinations. This results in a shorter exam time, increased patient throughput, decreased film costs, and a decrease in patient exposure.

2. A *100 or 105 mm photospot camera* can reduce film cost and patient exposure even more. This device also allows rapid filming of such dynamic events as swallowing at rates approaching ten frames per second. The time lag from the depression of the foot pedal or hand switch until the actual filming takes place is an order of magnitude shorter in using a photospot camera than it is in using a spot film device (up to 700 msec.).

3. A *non-silver halide film recording system* affords the ultimate in exposure and film cost reduction. One readily available and reasonably priced system is a high-resolution video tape machine (U-Matic, S-VHS, or other similar types) connected to the image intensifier. Videotape systems also afford a very high frame rate for recording swallowing studies, such as modified barium swal-

lows. Care must be taken to match the bandwidth to the imaging system, which usually precludes the use of consumer-type machines. In addition, consumer machines cannot record the typical high line rate TV images ($>1,000$) found in high-resolution image chains. Their greatest use may come in the field of medical education, where an examination may be recorded and then reviewed by the resident and responsible attending physician in order to clarify certain points in technique without subjecting the patient to further exposure. Digital-based recording systems are currently available. These also greatly decrease patient dose and allow editing of the obtained images (with window width and level controls similar to CT). Similarly, edge enhancement and other algorithms may be applied to the acquired data, allowing image manipulation leading to greater diagnostic accuracy.

Even as a first-year resident, one should be familiar with all the basic features of a flouoroscopy unit—turning on the generator, selecting both the fluoroscoping and filming kVp, selecting focal spot size, and choosing between phototiming and a manual technique. In addition, one should know how to insert and remove cassettes, insure that the grid is in place and that all the collimators and shutters are optimally opened, and that the area viewed during fluoroscopy is actually filmed. Although these are thought of as the responsibilities of the technologist, the resident should still possess this basic knowledge.

Additionally, if a resident learns how to load and unload cassettes (easily done with daylight film processor systems), an emergency exam can be significantly expedited even in the absence of a technologist. It cannot be overemphasized what a valuable (but altogether underutilized) resource technologists and/or supervisory personnel can be in learning these basics.

Single vs. Double Contrast

In our department a double contrast study is the rule unless it is contraindicated. In esophageal studies, the pure double contrast examination (which is done upright) does not afford evaluation of esophageal motor function. Therefore, in patients with suspected motility disturbances, it must be combined with or replaced by a recumbent single contrast exam. In addition, the upright positioning helps reduce a hiatal hernia, making their detection more difficult. Webs, rings, and other esophageal narrowings are better demonstrated with a solid column technique because of the better distention obtained while recumbent. In cases of suspected obstruction, a trial of a small amount of single contrast barium is warranted. Suspected foreign body obstructions, T-E fistulae, and achalasia all warrant special techniques that will be described in the following sections.

In patients with known or suspected gastric outlet obstruction, a single contrast study should be performed. The administration of gas-forming granules into a potentially closed system (lower esophageal sphincter closed proximally and obstruction distally) raises the possiblilty of perforation and therefore should be avoided.

All of our small bowel enemas are done in double contrast unless, during the filling phase, fluoroscopy reveals dilution by retained fluid. When excess fluid is encountered, the barium is diluted with sufficient water to decrease its concentration from 80 to 40 percent (adding one part water to one part barium). The exam is then continued as a single contrast enema.

In the colon, suspected obstruction is an indication for a single contrast exam. In cases of suspected diverticulitis, either a single or double contrast exam may be performed. The advantage of single contrast is that the thinner, less viscous barium may more readily fill diverticula, sinus tracts, or fistulae, thereby adding significant diagnostic information. The advantage of double contrast is that of detection of other mucosal abnormalities that may be present. The argument that double contrast exams create too much intraluminal pressure is only partly true. The mean pressures developed during both exams are the same. However, the peak pressures exerted, although transiently, are greater in the double contrast exam. Therefore, if a double contrast enema is performed, great care must be taken in the use of the air insufflation bulb, and only slow gentle squeezes of the insufflator used.

The role of the double contrast enema in the elderly patient is subject to an ongoing debate. If the patient is ambulatory, and if there is no strict contraindication for the type of physical activity necessary to perform the exam, then a double contrast exam is feasible. However, the principal advantage of the double contrast exam—finding diminutive polyps—may not be of great clinical significance in the elderly, considering the slow growth rate of the polyp versus the life expectancy of the patient. Therefore, the decision to use the double contrast technique in the elderly patient should be based on the unique set of facts for that individual patient.

Water Soluble Contrast vs. Barium

The two principal indications for the use of water soluble contrast are cases of suspected perforation and cases in which immediate surgery is planned and the presence of retained barium would complicate the surgery. The latter usually occurs during emergency "barium" enemas.

The use of water soluble contrast entails many compromises. First, it is not sufficiently radio-opaque. Studies have shown that a high percentage of perforations are missed on examinations performed solely with water soluble contrast. Therefore, it is strongly recommended (especially in the upper GI tract) that, if a water soluble study shows no evidence of a perforation, that it immediately be followed by a conventional single contrast barium examination. Second, Gastrografin and other similar agents do not sufficiently coat the mucosa. Therefore, important radiographs, such as the LPO spot film of the duodenal bulb, cannot demonstrate pathology on their nondependent surface. Third, conventional ionic contrast is markedly hypertonic. This causes considerable dilution of the contrast in the GI tract distal to the esophagus by causing fluid to shift into the extravascular compartment (intestinal lumen). This fluid shift also causes increased distention of the GI tract, which is theoretically, if not practically, contraindicated in cases of obstruction. Nonionic contrast may have theoretic advantages over the hyperosmolar ionic contrasts, but they are significantly more expensive, especially considering the large amounts often needed for these examinations. Fourth, the resultant distention from hypertonic contrast can increase peristaltic activity, which again may be contraindicated in cases of obstruction. Fifth, it should not be used in patients in whom aspiration or a T-E fistula is suspected. Water soluble (ionic) contrast in the lungs is very irritating and may cause a chemical pneumonitis. In addition, the hypertonicity noted above may cause non-cardiogenic pulmonary edema.

In the colon the decreased visibility of the contrast is problematic, particularly when looking for small fistulae (especially colovesical with dilution of the extravasated contrast within the urine-filled bladder). The hypertonicity may result in some dilution due to fluid shifts, but usually not to a clinically significant degree in the limited amount of time required to perform the examination. One advantage of this hypertonicity is that the influx of fluid may help clear the colon in cases of fecal impaction.

Examining Females of Childbearing Age

All females past the age of menarche are potentially pregnant. Therefore, the question "Is there any chance at all that you are pregnant?" should be asked of all menstruating females. Contrary to popular belief, upper socioeconomic classes are *not* immune to teenage pregnancy. The embarassment of a young, innocent patient is worthwhile compared with the risk of irradiating a pregnant woman. Ask the question yourself and do not depend on the patient reading a placard in the waiting room or on the door to the examining room (the patient may be preoccupied and not notice them). Ultimately, you are responsible for the radiation given to a patient.

Ask the question before every exam. In one instance, I received a negative response from a patient being evaluated for a pelvic mass. The barium enema confirmed the presence of a small mass. Three days later she returned for a small bowel series as part of her further work-up. After starting the exam, without again asking her the question, she told me, "By the way, you know that I just found out I am pregnant." Obviously, even in a three-day interval, circumstances may change.

The case of an accidentally irradiated pregnant female must be handled in an individualized manner and lies outside the scope of this handbook—except to say that the proverbial ounce of prevention is worth much more than the pound of cure.

How to Use Glucagon

It has been demonstrated that the intravenous administration of small doses of glucagon aids in the performance and accuracy of the double contrast UGI series. By lowering the tone of the GI tract smooth muscle and decreasing peristalsis and emptying, the stomach can be better examined. However, this must be balanced against the time and expense of IV administration, possible allergic and other side effects of the medication, and now—in the age of HIV infections—the risk of accidental exposure of the examiner.

In the examination of the esophagus and small bowel, there is almost no indication for glucagon's use. However, its greatest use is found in aiding the performance of the barium enema. By decreasing the mean intracolonic pressures developed during a barium enema, as well as decreasing the severity of spasmodic contractions, glucagon may allow the successful completion of an otherwise incomplete exam. However, reflux through the ileocecal valve becomes more common. This leads to possible compromise of the exam in at least two different ways: first, optimal distention may be lost secondary to the reflux of air into the small intestine; and second, refluxed barium in the ileum may overlap and obscure detail in the colon, especially in the sigmoid or a low-lying (ptotic) transverse colon.

When examining a patient who is S/P Billroth II (partial gastrectomy with gastrojejunostomy), glucagon is a necessity to slow gastric emptying through the wide-open anastomosis.

The dosages used are usually 0.1 to 0.2 mg IV for the routine UGI series; 0.3 mg IV for the post-operative stomach; and 1.0 mg IV for the routine colon exam. When used in the hospitalized patient, a progress note documenting its use should be placed in the chart. This may prevent a series of tests and consultations for the patient's otherwise unexplained hyperglycemia. The contraindications for its use include allergy to glucagon, known or suspected pheochromocytoma, insulinoma, and difficult-to-control ("brittle") diabetes mellitus.

Barium Enema Preparation

Adequate preparation of the colon should remove all particulate fecal material and leave little or no fluid residua. Various agents or combinations of agents have been proposed for this purpose, yet no single one stands out as so superior that it can supplant the others. The agents can be classified as electrolyte-balanced colon lavage solution; osmotic cathartics; irritant or contact cathartics; enemas and suppositories.

The advantages of the first agent (balanced electrolyte colonic lavage) are rapid onset of action, lack of significant intestinal cramping, lack of electrolyte disturbance post catharsis, and simplicity. Its disadvantages are nausea and vomiting (due to gastroparesis from the rapid ingestion of large amounts of chilled fluid) and large amounts of residual fluid in the colon. The latter may markedly interfere with barium coating. Also, decreased patient compliance is a problem due to the solution's "taste" and the need to ingest about four liters in a few hours. It has been advocated to use metaclopromide and bisacodyl tablets to decrease the gastroporesis and ensure the evacuation of residual fluid. This obviously complicates the otherwise simple nature of the preparation and adds to the cost, already the highest of all the alternatives.

Most other single-agent preparations have been found unsatisfactory and, therefore, commercial kits with up to three different components are marketed. These usually include an osmotic cathartic (such as magnesium citrate), a p.o. contact colon irritant (bisacodyl tablets or cascara derivative liquid), and a suppository or enema. These theoretically act by causing an osmotic influx of fluid into the small bowel and colon, and then subsequently emptying the right and the left colons with the additional agents.

Obviously the proper order and timing of the use of these agents needs a cooperative and comprehending patient. Some of the agents may cause abdominal cramps. The osmotic cathartics may be contraindicated in patients with decreased cardiac and/or renal function, due to their high sodium or magnesium content. One of the commercially available cascara-based cathartics comes dissolved in an ethanol base. This would be contraindicated in patients with pancreatitis and also counts as a carbohydrate exchange for diabetic patients.

A useful adjunct to these preparations is the administration of tap water enemas until clear, in the radiology department under the direct supervision of a trained technlogist. After a clear return is obtained, a minimum of one hour is needed to allow for water resorption before a double contrast barium enema may be performed. Unfortunately, few hospitals and offices have the necessary resources to implement such a program.

Of course the decision to use alternative cleansing regimens, or no preparation at all, can and should always be made with the patient's overall medical condition in mind. The patient's referring physician should always be contacted whenever there is doubt as to how to proceed.

Contraindications to Compression

Although graded compression is an extremely important part of the single contrast examination, its use is sometimes contraindicated or must be sharply curtailed. In severely osteopenic patients or patients with recent rib fractures, attempts to compress the fundus and high body of the stomach or the splenic flexure must be very limited so that rib fractures do not occur or are not exacerbated. In patients with an acute duodenal ulcer or severely inflamed or ischemic bowel, marked compression has been reported to result in perforation of the already diseased bowel. Patients with an abdominal aortic aneurysm should have limited compression performed for similar reasons. Marked splenomegaly, either neoplastic or inflammatory, also should limit or contraindicate the use of compression. Lastly, the recent post-operative patient cannot have pressure exerted on or near an incision lest the wound reopen. Patients with a decreased platelet count should be spared aggressive manipulation with the compression paddle.

Help and How to Get It

The best time to get help is *before* it is needed. Review all available and pertinent clinical information before starting a procedure. Plan what you are going to do and how you are going to do it. Be flexible if things don't go according to your plan. In most studies you can usually pause and reflect before proceeding anew. In the double contrast UGI series, speed is an important component of the successful exam (especially if no glucagon has been administered).

If the problem is technical in nature, ask your technologist for help. Especially in teaching hospitals, technologists may have had years more of experience than the junior resident who needs their help. A more senior resident, or the radiologist in charge of GI fluoroscopy, is another (and, hopefully, easily accessible) source of help. Obviously, this handbook has been prepared to help fill the void that has been perceived in teaching fluoroscopy.

The Recently Post-Operative Patient

Besides limiting the use of compression, the post-operative patient may have very slow or absent peristalsis. This is especially problematic following esophagectomies (partial or complete). Therefore, the head of the table should be elevated to decrease the risk of aspiration, but without raising it so high that the patient may slide off the table. The patient should have someone in attendance in the room at all times.

After stasis of contents in the esophagus and/or the stomach is noted and the exam completed, some consideration should be given to the removal of the contrast so that it cannot be regurgitated or refluxed and then aspirated.

Various compromises in patient positioning must be made in patients with various tubes, drains, and incisions that may limit a patient's mobility.

Post-Evacuation Film and the Barium Enema

There definitely is a role for post-evacuation films as a part of both single and double contrast barium enemas. In a BE with a feces-filled colon on the filled films, the post-evacuation film can assess the retention of both barium and stool. If only a small or no fecal residua remains following evacuation, the colon can be refilled and re-examined at that time, sparing the patient a return visit to the radiology department following a repeat bowel cleansing. In addition, the post-evacuation film aids in the differentiation of a spastic area of narrowing from a fixed stricture or other lesion (see also: **How to Use Glucagon**).

Because the intraluminal pressure during evacuation exceeds both the normal basal pressure of the colon and that developed during filling of the colon, diverticula, sinus tracts, fistulae, and other forms of possible extravasation from the colon are readily filled. The post-evacuation film helps document their presence.

Reports have indicated that the distention achieved during a double contrast enema may obliterate the mucosal and submucosal edematous changes seen in ischemic disease. (The same phenomena may theoretically occur in inflammatory bowel disease as well.) The use of the post-evacuation film may therefore be of use in these situations.

Lastly, the effects of an extrinsic mass on the colon may be more readily ascertained when the collapsed bowel drapes over the mass—rather than in the distended state when the air helps push the wall opposite the lesion away from the pathology.

Timing of Spot Films and Overheads

As a general rule, end expiration is the optimal phase in which to obtain spot films during a barium enema. The higher position of the diaphragm allows elongation of the flexure and less overlapping of the segments. Also, when patients take a deep breath and try to hold it, their whole body may shake, degrading the film with their marked inspiratory effort. A "dress rehearsal" of quiet breath-holding may be of help before proceeding with the exam.

Occasionally a duodenal bulb, hard to spot without overlapping loops of bowel, may best be seen in either a mid-inspiratory or mid-expiratory phase. This should be ascertained during fluoroscopic evaluation and the patient instructed to hold her or his breath at this optimal level.

Reporting of Examinations

When the examination is finished, the films should be viewed immediately to determine if they are technically adequate and if additional views are needed. At this time, a progress note with a preliminary report should be written in the chart. Additional comments in this note may document the use of glucagon or other medications. If pathology has been documented that needs immediate attention, a phone call to the proper personnel should be made and then documented in the chart.

A second viewing should be performed after the entire fluoroscopy schedule has been completed. This allows a more careful, unhurried look at the films. At this time the final, official report should be generated. If it conflicts with the preliminary, the contradiction should be noted in the report and the referring physician contacted to alert him or her to the changes.

A report should include the anatomic nature of the exam (UGI, SB, for example), the technique used (single contrast, double contrast, water soluble), as well as a complete review of what was seen. Pertinent negatives should be included so that the clinician knows that the particular clinical question has been addressed. Radiographic findings should be reported separately from their analysis. Recommendations for further clinical correlation and/or diagnostic imaging procedures should be included; but they should be worded appropriately so that the clinician's hands are not bound. All reports should have a concise conclusion that is directed at the clinical problem. A *Sample Report* is included in Appendix II.

The Patient with Heart Disease

In general, patients with most forms of heart disease do not need special handling. Patients with remote MI's or who are S/P CABG do not need any special precautions. A patient with a history of a recent MI should probably have a single contrast UGI, since it entails much less turning and patient manipulation compared to a double contrast examination. A BE should only be done if absolutely necessary, since the colonic distention and subsequent vagal stimulation may be deleterious. A period of six weeks should be considered the minimum interval for less-pressing situations.

Patients with a known diseased heart valve (MVP, AS, etc.) or a prosthetic valve do not need antibiotic prophylaxis even prior to a BE. Although bacteremia has been reported following both single and double contrast BEs, it is not thought to be severe or long-lasting enough to necessitate antibiotic usage. In addition, the bacterial flora introduced into the bloodstream from a BE are not those usually implicated in endocarditis.

The Recently Biopsied Patient

The timing of a post-biopsy examination depends on the type of biopsy and how it was obtained. A fiber-optic endoscope or colonoscope has a narrow instrument channel that limits the type of biopsy forceps used. These smaller instruments do not usually permit a very deep biopsy and, therefore, a barium exam may follow immediately (unless the patient's pharynx is still anesthetized with the associated risk of aspiration).

If a rigid prostoscope or sigmoidoscope has been used, the depth of biopsy may be much greater and a seven-day interval recommended before barium is administered.

The HIV Positive Patient

Patients with HIV infection should be handled in the same manner as any patient with an infectious disease. If there is any risk of contamination by bodily fluids, then rubber gloves should be worn. If large-scale contact is anticipated, then a gown as well as gloves should be used. If an aerosol spray from coughing, sneezing, or vomiting is antipicated, then protective eyewear and perhaps even a hood should also be used.

In all other cases, universal precautions should be used. Therefore, while inserting or manipulating any intestinal or rectal tube—as well as during the insertion of an IV line or the parenteral administration of medications—gloves should be worn.

Types of Barium

In the following chapters, the following definitions of barium will be used:

High-Density Barium:	150 to 250 percent w/v
Medium-Density Barium:	72 to 100 percent w/v
Low-Density Barium:	36 to 50 percent w/v
Very-Low-Density Barium:	15 to 20 percent w/v

Patient Positioning and Terminology

Strictly speaking, the position of the patient is named in regards to that portion of the patient closest to the imaging receptor. However, in most fluoroscopy units, the tube is under the table and the image intensifier or spot film device over the table—the reverse of the conventional overhead film set-up. In order to avoid confusion in switching terminologies for fluoroscopy and overheads (although the patient has not moved), I have adopted the terminology of the overhead film, with the positions named in reference to the table top (whether horizontal or vertical). Thus, a patient lying on his back, with the right side turned up, is in the **LPO** ⊗. Positioning charts are in Appendix III.

In the following chapters, the use of left and right on the fluoro screen refers to a patient in the anatomic position viewed on the screen. Therefore, "to the left of the spine" refers to the patient's left, or the viewer's right. When the patient is in a prone or prone oblique position, then "left" refers to the viewer's left. Referring to the line drawings should obviate any uncertainty.

Chapter 1

PHARYNX AND ESOPHAGUS–ROUTINE

PHARYNGOGRAM

RAPID SEQUENCE SWALLOWING STUDY

ESOPHAGRAM—SINGLE CONTRAST

ESOPHAGRAM—DOUBLE CONTRAST

PHARYNGOGRAM

PRELIMINARY FILMS: **UPRIGHT AP** ⊕, **LATERAL** OF THE NECK (soft-tissue techniques) [The patient should hold sandbags in her/his hands to lower the shoulders.]

CONTRAST: HIGH-DENSITY BARIUM

OVERHEADS: NONE

1. Start with the table upright, and the patient in the **RIGHT LATERAL** 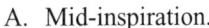 position. Have the patient take 1 swallow of barium and then spot the well-coated pharynx. The top of the film should be slightly above the level of the hard palate. Three exposures should be taken:

    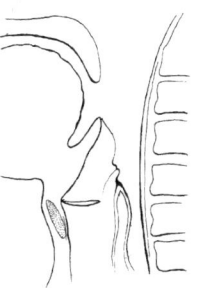

    A. Mid-inspiration.
    B. During a modified Valsalva maneuver.
    C. While phonating (long "e").
    Recoat the pharynx with another swallow of barium whenever necessary.

2. Turn the patient into the **AP** 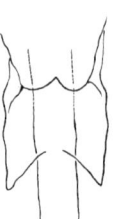 position. Recoat the mucosa with another swallow of the barium whenever necessary. The top of the film should be at the base of the tongue. Three exposures should be taken:
   A. Mid-inspiration.
   B. During a modified Valsalva maneuver.
   C. While phonating (long "e").

NOTES

1. Use a small focal spot for greater detail on the films.
2. A modified Valsalva is a forced expiration against a pinched-off nose and pursed lips.

RAPID SEQUENCE CERVICAL ESOPHAGRAM

PRELIMINARY FILMS: **SUPINE (AP)** ⊕ **AND LATERAL** FILMS OF THE SOFT TISSUES OF THE NECK

CONTRAST: MEDIUM-DENSITY BARIUM

WATER SOLUBLE CONTRAST (undiluted and unflavored with additives)

OVERHEADS: NONE

1. Place the table horizontal. Start with the patient in the **RIGHT LATERAL** ⊕ position. Have the patient swallow a small trial bolus of contrast. If no aspiration or extravasation of contrast is noted, proceed as below.

2. Film at the most rapid filming rate available. If videotape is available, use this as well.

3. Have the patient hold a barium bolus in the mouth until filming begins. Then have the patient swallow as rapidly as possible.

4. The first series of films should be obtained with the top of the film just above the level of the hard palate and the bottom below the level of the epiglottis. The fluoroscopy tower should be held still and not panned during the swallow. The barium should flow by a stationary recording set-up.

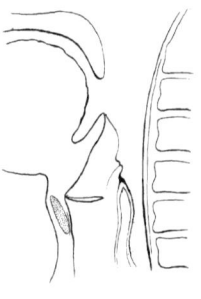

5. A second barium bolus should be administered and swallowed. For this swallow, the fluoroscopic image should include the top of the epiglottis and extend inferiorly. Again the fluoroscopy tower should not move during imaging.

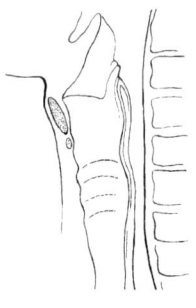

6. The patient should be placed in the **PRONE PA** (⊕) position for a frontal projection. Alternatively, the **SUPINE AP** (⊕) position may be used if necessary. The top of the fluoroscopy image should include the oral cavity and the base of the tongue. Again, have the patient hold the bolus of barium in the mouth until the command to swallow is given (after filming begins).

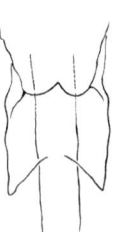

7. Examine the thoracic esophagus with either the single or double contrast techniques, as described on pages 28–31.

NOTES

1. Accurate positioning of the patient in a true lateral position is very important for properly examining swallowing. Care must be taken to insure that the mandibles are properly superimposed over one another. The cervical spine should be seen in the lateral and not oblique projection at the same time.

2. Step 7, above, is included because many complaints of dysphagia referable to the neck are really secondary to more distal pathology. Patients are very often poor localizers of their pathology. Dysmotility seen in the pharyngoesophageal region may also be secondary to more distal pathology.

ESOPHAGUS–SINGLE CONTRAST

PRELIMINARY FILM: **AP** ⊕ BUCKY CHEST

CONTRAST: LOW-DENSITY BARIUM

OVERHEADS: **RAO** ⊘, **PA** ⊕, AND **RIGHT LATERAL** ⊕ WHILE THE PATIENT IS RAPIDLY DRINKING

1. Start with the table horizontal and the patient in **RAO** ⊘. Have the patient swallow one small bolus of barium. Follow the bolus from the oral cavity to the stomach. If there is good mucosal coating, obtain collapsed (mucosal relief) overlapping films of the entire length of the thoracic esophagus. The esophagus should project just to the right of, and without overlapping, the spine.

2. In the same position **RAO** (⊘) have the patient drink rapidly and spot the esophagus in overlapping segments. The gastroesophageal junction should be spotted after the patient performs a Valsalva maneuver (ask the patient to strain as if moving their bowels) to accentuate a hiatal hernia.

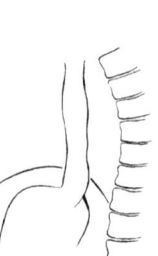

3. Repeat step 2 in the **RIGHT LATERAL** ⊕ projection, omitting the Valsalva maneuver. In this position the esophagus projects anterior to the spine.

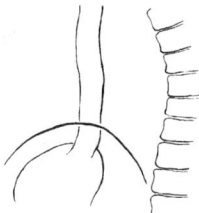

4. Repeat step 2 in the **PRONE PA** (⊖) projection, omitting the Valsalva maneuver. In this position the esophagus projects over the spine in the midline, only curving away as it approaches the diaphragm.

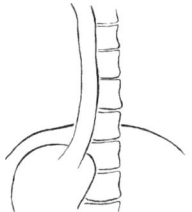

NOTE

1. If a hiatal hernia or stricture is suspected but not well visualized, or if dysphagia is not well explained on the original study, an iced barium preparation is recommended. This may be made by mixing equal amounts of high-density barium (250 percent w/v) with cracked ice. The ice cold mixture will cause a marked decrease in the primary peristalsis, allowing better visualization of relative narrowings and accentuating dysmotility.

ESOPHAGUS–DOUBLE CONTRAST

PRELIMINARY FILM: AP ⊕ BUCKY CHEST

CONTRAST: HIGH-DENSITY BARIUM
LOW-DENSITY BARIUM

OVERHEADS: NONE

1. Start with the table horizontal and the patient in the **RAO** ⊗ projection. Have the patient swallow one small sip of the high-density barium. Follow the bolus from the oral cavity to the stomach. Spot the collapsed mucosal relief films of the entire esophagus in overlapping segments. The esophagus should project just to the right of, and without overlapping, the spine (on the same side as the stomach).

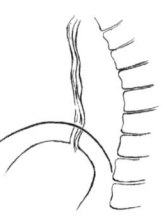

2. Bring the table to the full upright position. Place the patient in the **LPO** ⊗ position. Have the patient swallow the gas-forming granules with no more than 15 cc of water. Immediately following the ingestion of the granules, have the patient very rapidly gulp the high-density barium. As the esophagus becomes air-filled and distended, spot the well-coated esophagus in overlapping segments. The esophagus should project to the left of

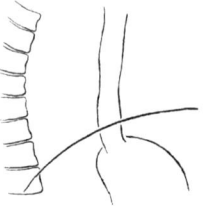

the spine without being superimposed on that structure.

3. Return the table to the horizontal position. Place the patient in the **RAO** ⊘ position. Have the patient rapidly drink the lower-density single contrast barium. Spot the well-distended esophagus in overlapping segments. Have the patient strain (perform a Valsalva maneuver) and spot the gastroesophageal junction for a possible hiatal hernia. The position of the esophagus should be the same as in step 1.

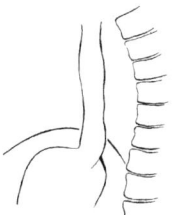

NOTES

1 If barium fills the esophagus more than air, and if there is an air-fluid level present, wait for the air-fluid level to descend. Spot the air-filled esophagus just proximal to (above) the descending air-fluid level.

2. The rapid and repetitive swallowing of the barium superimposes peristaltic waves upon one another, leading to atonia of the esophagus and subsequent excellent distention.

Chapter 2

PHARYNX AND ESOPHAGUS–SPECIAL

OBSTRUCTION

PERFORATION

ACHALASIA

VARICES

FOREIGN BODY

T-E FISTULA

"PULL-THROUGH"

ESOPHAGOJEJUNOSTOMY

COLON INTERPOSITION

CELESTINE TUBE

ESOPHAGEAL OBSTRUCTION

1. The techniques used in cases of esophageal obstruction vary as to the expected nature of the underlying pathology. Separate chapters exist to cover the obstructing foreign body (such as an impacted meat bolus), as well as achalasia.

2. In those cases in which a stricture—benign or malignant—is suspected, the routine examinations outlined elsewhere should be sufficient. It is always extremely important to start out with small amounts of barium and observe the flow through the esophagus; very often this will give sufficient information that the examination can be halted and the patient obtain immediate intervention. In other cases, the full diagnostic examination may then be performed. Not "flooding" the esophagus and obscuring detail, and not placing the patient at risk for aspiration (with the increased volume of barium and retained secretions proximal to the obstruction) remain the very highest priorities in examining the obstructed esophagus.

ESOPHAGEAL PERFORATION

PRELIMINARY FILM: **AP** ⊕ BUCKY CHEST

CONTRAST: WATER SOLUBLE CONTRAST (30% IODINATED)

OVERHEADS: **SUPINE (AP)** ⊕, **RIGHT LATERAL** ⊕ CHEST (IF EXTRAVASATION)

1. With the table horizontal, place the patient in the **RIGHT LATERAL** ⊕. Administer 10 cc of water soluble contrast via a catheter-tip syringe and have the patient swallow. Observe closely for possible aspiration. If present, switch to barium as contrast agent. (See *Notes* below.)

2. If no aspiration or extravasation is seen, have the patient drink larger amounts of water soluble contrast through a straw and spot the distended esophagus in overlapping segments as it projects anterior to the spine.

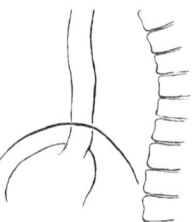

PHARYNX AND ESOPHAGUS—SPECIAL

3. With the patient in the **RAO** ⊘ position, spot the entire esophagus in overlapping segments while the patient is drinking. The esophagus should project to the right of the spine without actually overlapping it.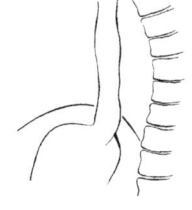

4. With the patient in the **PA** ⊕ **(PRONE)** position spot the entire esophagus in overlapping segments while the patient is drinking. The esophagus will overlie the spine in this position, with only the GE junction projecting to the right.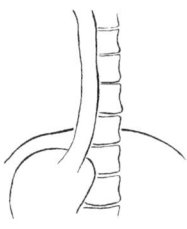

NOTES

1. If no perforation is seen, repeat with low-density barium as per the single contrast esophagram protocol.

2. If aspiration is noted upon swallowing, and if perforation or fistulization to the tracheobronchial tree is present, an alternative agent is nonionic contrast. At the time of this book's preparation, the use of nonionics for this purpose was not FDA approved. Before proceeding with its use, please check with legal counsel, or other authority concerning any liability arising from nonapproved usage of contrast approved for other purposes.

ACHALASIA

PRELIMINARY FILMS: **PA** ⊕, **LATERAL** CHEST

CONTRAST: HIGH-DENSITY BARIUM

OVERHEADS: **PA** ⊕ CHEST (UPRIGHT)

1. Start with the patient in the **LPO** ⊗ with the table upright. Have the patient drink 10 to 15 cc of the high-density barium.

2. Watch the barium "percolate" through the food and fluid-filled esophagus, which may project to the left of the spine or overlap it, depending on the degree of dilatation and resultant tortuosity.

3. As the barium outlines the narrowed subdiaphragmatic esophagus, spot the GE junction as it lies just to the left of the spine.

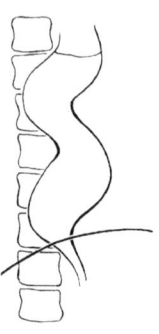

NOTES

1. If no air-fluid level is observed on upright fluoroscopy, and if no esophageal narrowing or delayed emptying is seen, then proceed with a routine esophagram.

2. If a classic deformity of the distal esophagus is seen, the exam is usually terminated. The presence of large amounts of retained food and fluid prevent adequate evaluation of the more proximal esophageal mucosa.

3. Unlike conventional obstructions, the achalasia esophagus will partially empty itself spontaneously. The use of a small amount of barium does not usually place the patient at increased risk of aspiration from the exam.

ESOPHAGEAL VARICES

The examination for esophageal varices is usually a part of a more complete UGI series. Therefore, the techniques described below should be considered modifications of the more extensive techniques outlined in the appropriate UGI or esophagram sections. The principles upon which these modifications are based are those that will enhance filling and engorgement of the variciosities. These include:

1. *Quiet respiration.* Marked changes in the intrathoracic pressure may lead to emptying or decreased filling of the varices.

2. *Stoppage of esophageal peristalsis.* Any contraction of the esophageal wall will decrease variceal distention. Therefore, after adequate coating is obtained with an initial swallow of high-density barium, no swallowing at all is allowed. Within a short period of time, the varices will redistend. A small basin may be provided into which the patient may expectorate, instead of swallowing his saliva.

3. *Proper positioning.* Visualization of varices is enhanced with the patient in the **RAO** ⊗ position (prone oblique) with the table horizontal. This promotes filling of the varices from the splenic vein.

RETAINED ESOPHAGEAL FOREIGN BODY

PRELIMINARY FILMS:

   A. **LATERAL** OF THE NECK with low kVp for soft tissue technique

   B. **PA** ⊖ and **LEFT LATERAL** ⊕ OF THE CHEST

CONTRAST: HIGH-DENSITY BARIUM

            OTHER: COTTON BALLS SOAKED IN HIGH-DENSITY BARIUM AND THEN FLUFFED UP

OVERHEADS: NONE

IMPACTED FOOD OR OBSTRUCTING FOREIGN BODY

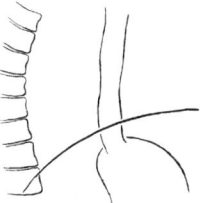

1. Start with the table upright and the patient in the **LPO** ⊗ position. Administer 5 cc of high-density barium in a small medicine cup or via a catheter-tip syringe. Have the patient swallow and follow the barium distally until the obstructing foreign body is outlined. Spot the obstruction. If no obstructing lesion is seen, then proceed as a routine single contrast esophogram.

NOTES

1. Patients with an obstructing foreign body usually are drooling and have a fluid-filled esophagus proximal to the impaction. The use of a small amount of high-density barium allows it to pass through this pool of secretions without adding signifi-

cantly to its volume. The high-density barium "sinks" to the bottom without becoming so dilute that the offending material is missed. Lower-density barium may not "sink" as readily and may become too dilute to adequately visualize the foreign body.

2. A post–foreign body removal exam is strongly recommended to determine the underlying cause of the impaction.

RETAINED CHICKEN OR FISH BONE

1. Start with the table upright and the patient in the **RIGHT LATERAL** ⊕ position. Administer 5 cc of high-density barium via a small medicine cup or syringe. Have the patient swallow the bolus. Spot the well-coated, well-distended pharynx during a modified Valsalva maneuver (expiration through pursed lips with the nose pinched).

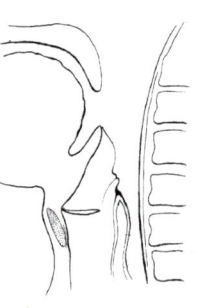

2. Repeat step 1 with the patient in the **AP** ⊕ position.

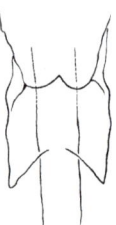

3. If no foreign body is identified, then repeat steps 1 and 2 using the barium-soaked cotton balls.

NOTES

1. The emphasis of the fish bone study is on the pharynx with its vallecula and pyriform sinus recesses, since these are the most common sites for entrapment of linear foreign bodies.
2. The barium-soaked cotton ball is used as an adjunct so that one or more fibers may catch on the rough edge of a bone and remain there *post-swallowing* to render the lucent cartilaginous fish bone more apparent. Chicken bones are usually very well calcified and evident on the preliminary films.

TRACHEOESOPHAGEAL FISTULA

PRELIMINARY FILM: **AP** ⊕ CHEST

CONTRAST: MEDIUM-DENSITY BARIUM

OVERHEADS: **AP** ⊕, **LATERAL** CHEST

1. Place the patient on a horizontal table in the **RIGHT LATERAL** ⊕ position. Administer a small (5 cc) bolus of barium and observe its passage through the esophagus. Spot in overlapping segments the intrathoracic esophagus from the inlet to below the carina.

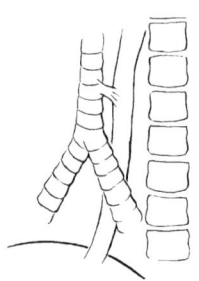

2. Repeat step 1 with larger boluses and then continuous drinking of barium if no aspiration or fistularization is seen. Spot the better-distended esophagus to the level of the carina. If the airway is still free of contrast, then proceed with a routine single contrast esophagram.

NOTES

1. Careful attention should be made to the route of filling of the tracheobronchial tree with barium. Observation under fluoroscopy should reveal whether the patient aspirated or the tracheobronchial tree filled through a fistula. Along with

pharyngeal swallowing studies, this is the exam in which videotape may play its largest role.

2. If the route of filling of the tracheobronchial tree was missed during the initial exam, and videotape or cine is not available for review, there is still a technique of salvaging the exam without repeating it. Place the image intensifier in its highest magnification mode (smallest field of view). Have the patient breathe deeply. Careful observation may reveal barium from the trachea transiting the fistula to enter the esophagus, or vice versa.

POST-ESOPHAGOGASTRECTOMY

PRELIMINARY FILMS: AP ⊕ BUCKY CHEST, AP ⊕ **(SUPINE)** ABDOMEN

CONTRAST: WATER SOLUBLE CONTRAST
MEDIUM-DENSITY BARIUM

OVERHEADS: **AP** ⊕ **(SUPINE), RAO** ⊘, **LAO** ⊘ OF THE ESOPHAGUS while drinking [If the patient cannot be placed in prone obliques, then **RPO** ⊘ and **LPO** ⊘ can be substituted.]

AP ⊕ **(SUPINE)** ABDOMEN

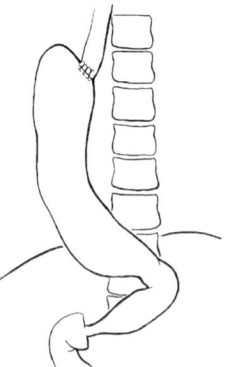

1. The head of the table should be elevated approximately 15 to 20 degrees, if well tolerated by the patient. If the patient is recently post-operative, he should be placed in the **RPO** ⊘ position. Have the patient swallow one small bolus of water soluble contrast (if the patient is immediately post-operative and extravasation is possible). Spot the esophagogastric anastamosis.

2. Steepen the obliquity, if the patient's condition and tubes and lines permit. Repeat the small swallow of water soluble contrast and spot the gastrotomy staple line.

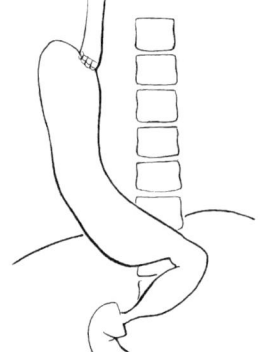

3. Place the patient in the **AP** ⊕ **(SUPINE)** position and examine the intrathoracic portion of the stomach.

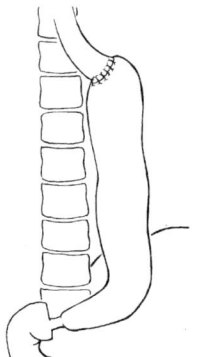

4. Turn the patient into the **LPO** ⊗ position to allow contrast to flow to the part of the pulled-through stomach that transits the diaphragm through the esophageal hiatus to enter the abdomen. Spot this segment if it fills.

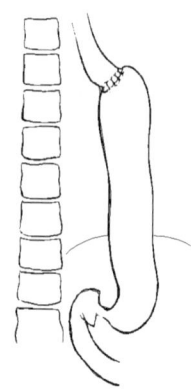

5. If no leak is seen during fluoroscopy and on the developed spot films, then proceed as follows.

6. With the table horizontal, place the patient in the **RAO** ⊗ position. Have the patient swallow a small amount of barium and spot the esophagogastric anastamosis.

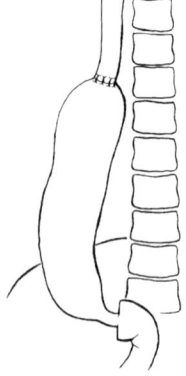

7. Place the patient in the **PA (PRONE)** position and have the patient continue drinking. Spot the esophagogastric anastamosis again.

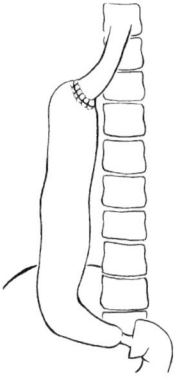

8. Turn the patient into the **LAO** and spot the gastrotomy staple line.

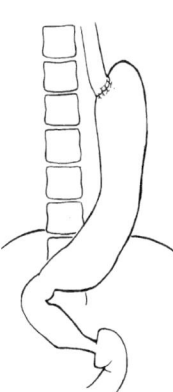

9. Place the patient in the **AP** ⊕ **(SUPINE)** position and examine the intrathoracic portion of the stomach.

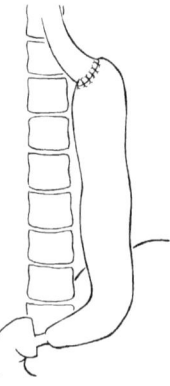

10. Turn the patient into the **LPO** ⊗ position to allow contrast to flow to the part of the pulled-through stomach that transits the diaphragm through the esophageal hiatus to enter the abdomen. Spot this segment if it fills.

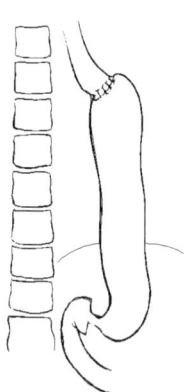

NOTES

1. If the patient is not immediately post-operative, then start with barium as in step 6.

2. If the esophageal remnant empties too rapidly for conventional spot filming, a rapid-sequence camera should be used to evaluate this segment as well as the anastamosis. If this is not available, the head of the table can be lowered. This may allow reflux of the contrast from the intrathoracic gastric rem-

nant into the esophageal remnant. This allows retrograde filling and visualization of the anastamosis. This must be done with great care since the risk of aspiration is high using this controlled reflux. Only experienced fluoroscopists should attempt this maneuver, and its risks must be balanced against the additional information gained by the technique.

3. Speak to the surgeon or know the exact details of the surgery performed. Many times there is a blind-ending gastric pouch adjacent to the anastamosis that may be misinterpreted as an area of extravasation.

4. An easy way of limiting the amount of contrast swallowed is to place 10 to 15 cc of contrast into a catheter-tip syringe and use this to gently introduce the contrast into the patient's mouth.

5. At the end of the procedure, the intrathoracic stomach should be checked for retained contrast. If present, consider using an NG tube to drain the residua. This should lower the patient's risk of aspiration after he leaves the Radiology Department flat on his back. Keeping the head of the stretcher elevated may also decrease this risk.

POST-ESOPHAGOJEJUNOSTOMY

PRELIMINARY FILM: **AP ⊕ (SUPINE)** UPPER ABDOMEN TO INCLUDE THE DIAPHRAGM

CONTRAST: WATER SOLUBLE CONTRAST, FOLLOWED BY MEDIUM-DENSITY BARIUM

OVERHEADS: **AP ⊕ (SUPINE), RPO ⊘ , LPO ⊘** IF RECENTLY POST-OP

PA ⊕ (PRONE), RAO ⊘ , LAO ⊘ IF NOT

1. Place the table horizontal. Place the patient in the **RPO ⊘** position. Have the patient swallow a small bolus of contrast. Follow this fluoroscopically through the esophagus, as it projects to the right of the spine, until the esophagojejunal anastamosis is traversed, probably to the right of the spine. Spot the anastamosis.

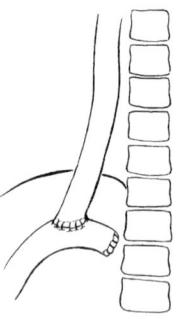

2. Turn the patient into the **LPO** ⊗ position. Repeat the swallow and spot the anastamosis again.

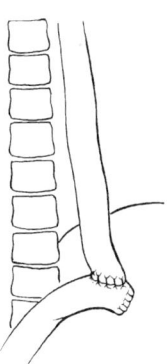

3. Turn the patient appropriately to fill the blind-ending jejunal pouch and spot this.

4. If no extravasation is seen during fluoroscopy and on the spot films, proceed with barium as the contrast agent and repeat steps 1 to 3.

5. If the patient is not recently postoperative, or if extravasation is not a concern after steps 1 to 4, then the examination should proceed with barium as the contrast agent. Spot the esophagus in overlapping segments in the **RAO** ⊗ position while the patient drinks barium.

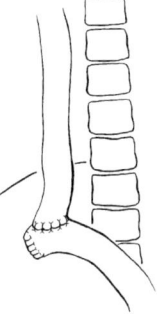

6. Turn the patient into the **RIGHT LATERAL** ⊕ and spot the well-distended esophagus in overlapping segments while the patient drinks barium.

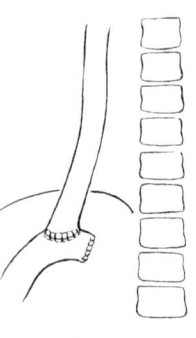

7. Turn the patient into the **PA** ⊕ **(PRONE)** position and spot the well-distended esophagus in overlapping segments while the patient drinks barium.

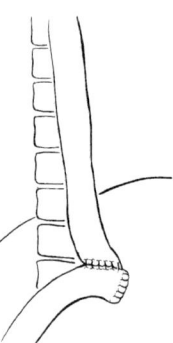

NOTES

1. Do not proceed with steps 5 to 7 if there is significant esophageal dysperistalsis. The sequelae of aspiration, even of relatively benign barium, may be too severe for a recently post-operative patient to tolerate.

2. A jejunal pouch may resemble localized extravasation. Sometimes the jejunum is doubled back upon itself and then opened to form a large reservoir. These and other variations of surgical techniques should be discussed with the referring surgeon prior to the performance of the exam to prevent any misinterpretation of the films.

POST-COLONIC INTERPOSITION

1. Proceed as if the patient has had an esophagogastrectomy ("pull-through") with the following caveats:
   A. The proximal anastamosis may be in the neck rather than in the thorax; therefore, the patient is at higher risk for aspiration. Consultation with the attending surgeon is recommended to evaluate the risk of aspiration of water soluble contrast versus the risk of extravasated barium in the neck and/or mediastinum.
   B. The interposed colonic segment is nonperistaltic. Extreme care must be taken to prevent delayed aspiration after the study has been completed and contrast remains in the colon. Attempts should be made to drain the contrast by carefully introducing an NG tube or using a previously placed tube.

C. The lower anastamosis (cologastric or even coloenteric) should be visualized and spotted as well. The exact position necessary to visualize this region cannot be predicted in advance due to the variations in anatomy and techniques used in the surgery. Close fluoroscopic monitoring of the procedure will give the answer.

CELESTINE TUBE IMPLANT STUDY

PRELIMINARY FILMS: **AP** ⊕ BUCKY CHEST

CONTRAST: WATER SOLUBLE CONTRAST (if recently placed or a perforation is suspected)

MEDIUM-DENSITY BARIUM (if tubal patency is to be checked, or if a T-E fistula is suspected)

OVERHEADS: **AP** ⊕ **(SUPINE), RPO** ⊗ **, LPO** ⊗

1. If the patient can tolerate it, raise the head of the table 15 to 20 degrees. Place the patient in a moderate **RPO** ⊗ so that the tube projects to the right of the spine. Have the patient swallow one small bolus of contrast and observe its flow. If there is no gross extravasation or obstruction, repeat the swallow and spot the upper esophageal-tube junction.

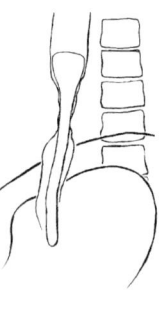

2. As contrast exits the tube, spot the lower esophageal-tube junction or the flow into the stomach.

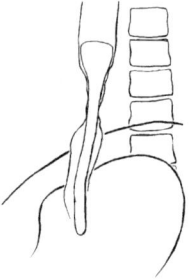

3. Turn the patient into the **LPO** ⊗ position so that the tube does not overlie the spine and repeat steps 1 and 2.

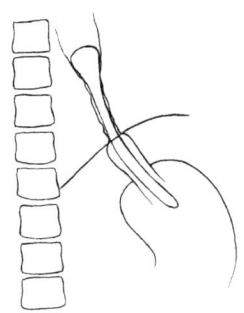

4. If the exam utilized water soluble contrast, and if no extravasation is seen in steps 1 to 3, then repeat with barium as the contrast.

NOTES

1. The table tilt aids in the prevention of reflux in the rigid, aperistaltic prosthetic tube. The use of a completely upright position of the patient would lead to too rapid emptying of the prosthesis and inadequate visualization of the esophagus.

2. At the proximal esophageal-tube junction, there is a wide flange that should prevent contrast leakage into the native diseased esophagus. If contrast leaks around this flange, additional spots should be obtained to look for extravasation or filling of a T-E fistula.

3. Some tubes have a similar but smaller flange at their lower end. Contrast may leak around this to enter the native esophagus in a retrograde manner. This may result in filling of a T-E fistula or extravasation, as noted above. In order to test for this possibility, the table may be placed either horizontally or even in a mild Trendelenburg position. Contrast in the stomach or distal esophagus may then be "refluxed" up to and around the lower flange. Because of the high risk of aspiration in this maneuver, it should only be attempted if the upper esophagus is clear of retained contrast and the examiner is ready to change the table tilt immediately if necessary. I recommend this maneuver be performed by those highly experienced in GI radiology and not by a novice.

4. As in other instances in which the amount of contrast to be used must be limited, a catheter-tip syringe may be used to introduce the correct amount into the patient's mouth.

Chapter 3

Stomach–Routine

Upper GI—Single Contrast
Upper GI—Double Contrast

UPPER GI SERIES–SINGLE CONTRAST

PRELIMINARY FILM: **AP ⊕ (SUPINE)** ABDOMEN

CONTRAST: LOW-DENSITY BARIUM

OVERHEADS: **AP ⊕ (SUPINE), RAO ⊗, RIGHT LATERAL ⊕, RPO ⊘, LPO ⊗** OF STOMACH, **PA ⊖ (PRONE)** FULL ABDOMEN

1. Place the table level and the patient in a **RAO ⊗** projection. Have the patient swallow a small bolus of barium and follow this fluoroscopically to the stomach. Spot, in overlapping segments, the collapsed, mucosal relief of the coated esophagus. The esophagus should project to the right of the spine, on the same side as the stomach.

   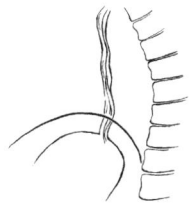

2. With the small amount of barium coating the gastric rugae, place a compression paddle underneath the patient and inflate the balloon to apply sufficient pressure to spread apart the folds and "see through" the barium. Spot the body (A), antrum (B), and duodenal bulb (C) and sweep (D). The bulb should not be superimposed upon the spine, although the descending portion of the sweep may be.

   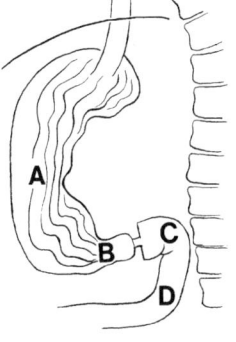

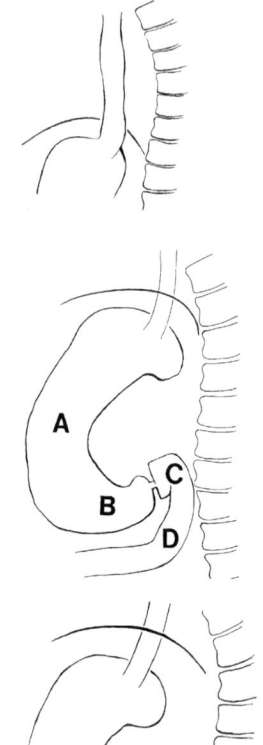

3. Have the patient rapidly drink large amounts of barium. Spot the fully-distended esophagus in overlapping segments. Have the patient strain (Valsalva maneuver), while the esophagus is fully distended, just prior to spotting the gastroesophageal junction.

4. Using the previously placed compression paddle, spot the fully-distended stomach and duodenum with adequate compression to see fold detail through the barium. Move the paddle to examine, fully both the body (A) and antrum, (B), as well as the bulb (C) and sweep (D).

5. Remove the compression paddle. Turn the patient into the **RIGHT LATERAL** ⊕. Spot the distal antrum, bulb, and sweep when they are fully distended. The descending duodenum should project just anterior to the spine.

6. Continue turning the patient into the **RPO** ⊘. Spot the mid-portion of the stomach, with particular attention to the lesser curvature. If the barium is too dense to see detail in the stomach, use the compression paddle on the anterior abdominal wall to aid in penetration. The mid-portion of the lesser curvature should be superimposed over the spine or just to the right of it.

    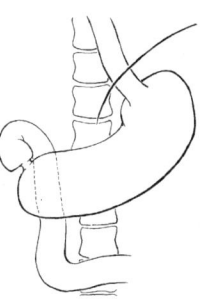

    A. With barium covering the GE junction, and while still in the **RPO** ⊘, have the patient strain (Valsalva) and watch to see if barium refluxes into the distal esophagus. Spot the superior extent of the reflux and make note of how promptly the refluxed material is cleared from the entire esophagus.

7. Turn the patient into the **AP** ⊕ **(SUPINE)** position. Spot the mid-portion of the stomach, which should be partially air-filled. The antrum will be superimposed over the spine, while the bulb and descending duodenum will be on the right, away from the stomach.

    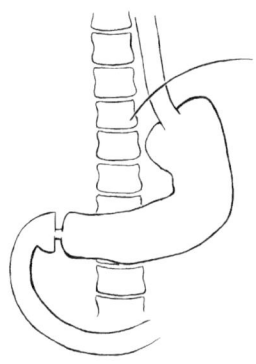

8. Turn the patient into the **LPO** ⊗ position and allow air to rise into the distal antrum and duodenal bulb. The patient should be positioned so that there is no overlapping of the bulb, either over the lesser curvature (overrotated) or over the descending duodenum (underrotated). Usually the bulb will project just to the left of the spine on the same side as the stomach. Spot the air-distended and well-coated antrum (A) and bulb (B) and sweep (C) at least twice.

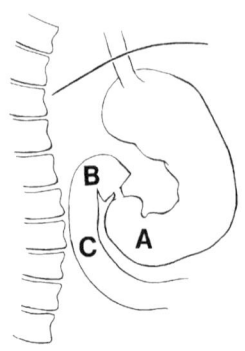

NOTES

1. Always start the examination with small sips of barium. It is much easier to give additional barium than it is to deal with excessive amounts to obtain good mucosal relief.

2. Do not spend too much time and use too much barium during the initial examination of the esophagus. You can always reexamine it with lots of barium at the end of the study.

3. Sometimes, at step 8, the bulb is not well coated with barium. If this occurs, turn the patient **AP** ⊕ **(SUPINE)** and then **RIGHT LATERAL** ⊕, to allow the bulb to refill with barium. As soon as this occurs, reposition the patient in the **LPO** ⊗ to obtain the spots.

4. Another frequently encountered problem at step 8 is that of a barium-filled bulb that does not allow good air contrast to be obtained. When this occurs, attempts to drain the excess barium should be made. The patient may be overrotated into the **LEFT LATERAL** ⊕ and the barium drained through the pylorus back into the antrum. Alternatively, the patient may be placed on his back in the **AP** ⊕ **(SUPINE)** position. This allows the barium to flow into the more posterior descending duodenum. A minimal degree of head-up table tilt may aid this maneuver. As soon as the excess barium is drained, the patient should be repositioned into the optimal **LPO** ⊗ to obtain the bulb air contrast spots.

UPPER GI SERIES–DOUBLE CONTRAST

PRELIMINARY FILM: **AP ⊕ (SUPINE)** ABDOMEN

CONTRAST: HIGH-DENSITY BARIUM
               LOW-DENSITY BARIUM

OVERHEADS: **PA ⊕ (PRONE)** ABDOMEN

1. Start with the table horizontal and the patient in the **RAO** ⊘ position. Have the patient swallow a small bolus of the high-density barium. Spot the collapsed, coated mucosal relief of the esophagus in overlapping segments. The esophagus should project to the right of the spine, on the same side as the stomach.

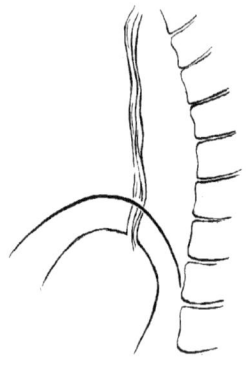

2. Place the compression paddle under the patient. Apply sufficient compression to "see through" the barium and visualize the rugal folds. Spot the gastric body (A) and antrum (B), as well as the duodenal bulb (C) and sweep (D) in overlapping segments. The bulb should not be superimposed upon the spine, although the descending portion of the sweep may be. Do not wait for the duodenum to fill if glucagon has

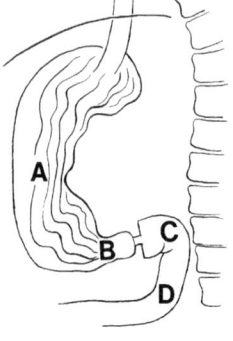

been previously administered. Proceed with the rest of the exam.

3. Turn the patient **AP** ⊕ **(SUPINE)** and bring the table to the full upright position.

4. Place the patient **LPO** ⊗. Have the patient swallow the gas-producing granules with 10 to 15 cc of water. Immediately follow the granules with very rapid gulping of the high-density barium. As the esophagus becomes air-filled and distended, take overlapping spot films of the well-coated esophagus, as it projects to the left of the spine, on the same side as the stomach.

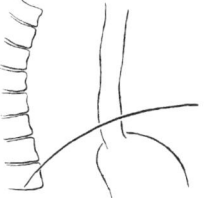

5. Turn the patient **PA** ⊕ **(PRONE)**, facing the table top, and lower the table to the horizontal plane.

6. Turn the patient quickly in the following sequence: **PA** ⊕ **(PRONE); LEFT LATERAL** ⊕; **AP** ⊕ **(SUPINE); LEFT LATERAL** ⊕; **PA** ⊕ **(PRONE); LEFT LATERAL** ⊕; **AP** ⊕ **(SUPINE); RIGHT LATERAL** ⊕; **PA** ⊕ **(PRONE); LEFT LATERAL** ⊕; ending in the **LPO** ⊗. This turning sequence places the right side down only once, to prevent

rapid emptying of the stomach and premature filling of the sweep, with possible overlapping of the stomach.

7. In the **LPO** ⊗ position, spot the distal half of the stomach which is air-filled and well-coated. The entire stomach should project to the left of the spine.

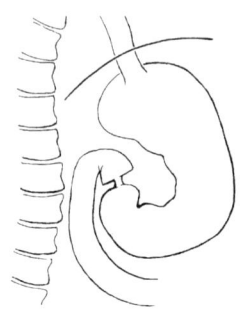

8. Turn the patient **AP** ⊕ **(SUPINE)**. Spot the distal half of the air-filled, well-coated stomach. The distal portion of the antrum should overlie the spine.

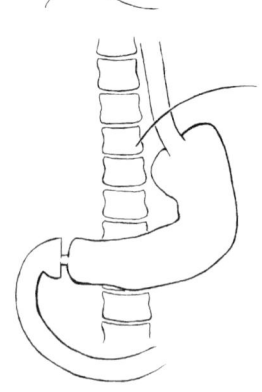

STOMACH—ROUTINE

9. Turn the patient into a shallow **RPO** ⊘. Spot the distal half of the lesser curvature as it projects just to the right of the spine.

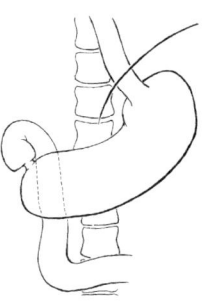

10. Turn the patient into the **RIGHT LATERAL** ⊕ position. Spot the air-filled fundus and proximal body of the stomach. They should project anterior to the spine. If possible, time the exposure so that the duodenal bulb and sweep are barium-filled at the same time.

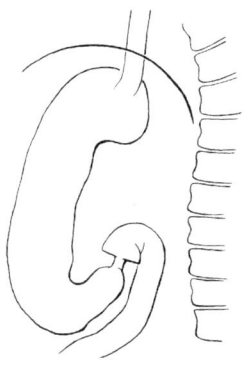

11. Turn the patient back into a medium **RPO** ⊘. Allow the barium to flow in a retrograde manner from the distal stomach to refill the previously air-filled fundus. As it flows along the proximal lesser curvature, spot this region with a thin barium pool being present. The more proximal to mid-lesser curvature should overlie the spine.

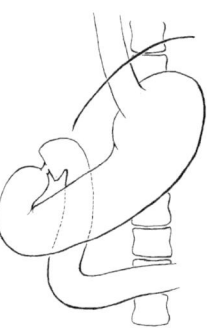

12. Turn the patient **AP** ⊕ **(SU-PINE)** and then into the **LEFT LATERAL** ⊕. Spot the distal antrum and bulb in an "end-on" projection. If the anterior wall of the distal antrum and bulb are not well seen, the patient may be overrotated into a very steep **LAO** ⊘ in order to better visualize this area. If too much barium is present in the distal body to allow sufficient visualization of the antrum, place the table head down 15 to 20 degrees.

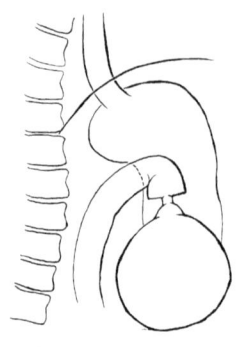

13. Turn the patient into the **LPO** ⊘. Spot the air-filled distal antrum (A), bulb (B), and (C) sweep at least twice. They should project to the left of the spine on the same side as the stomach. Care should be taken so that there is not much, if any, overlapping of the bulb on the lesser curvature or descending duodenum.

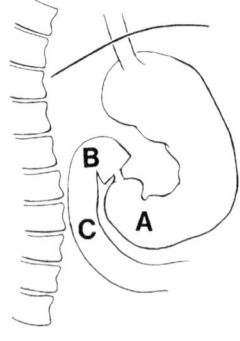

14. Place the patient **AP** ⊕ **(SU-PINE)** and bring the table to the full upright position.

15. Turn the patient **LPO** ⊗ and spot the air-filled fundus. The degree of obliquity should be one that eliminates overlapping of the undersurface of the fundus with the high-lesser curvature. In a very transverse stomach, this may not be feasible and an **RPO** ⊘ will be required to view the fundus well.

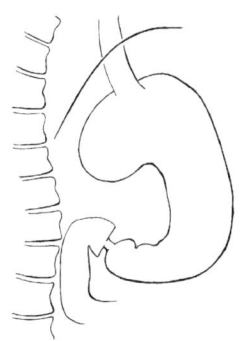

16. Turn the patient **PA** ⊕ **(PRONE)** facing the table and lower the table to the horizontal position.

17. Turn the patient into the **RAO** ⊗ position. Have the patient rapidly drink the dilute barium to fully distend the esophagus. Spot the distended esophagus in overlapping segments; it should project to the right of the spine. Spot the GE junction immediately following a Valsalva maneuver performed while the esophagus is still barium-filled.

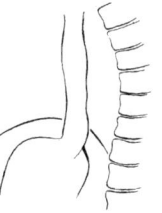

18. Turn the patient **AP** ⊕ **(SU-PINE)** and raise the table to the upright position. Turn the patient into the **LPO** ⊗ and use the compression device on the fluoro tower to compress the body (A), antrum (B), and bulb (C). Alternatively, the patient may be kept in the **RAO** ⊗ with the table horizontal, and compression spot films can be obtained with the paddle inserted underneath the patient.

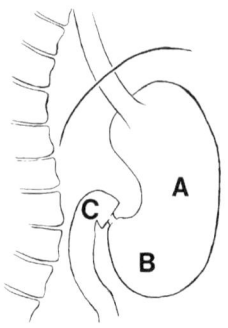

NOTES

1. Use glucagon 0.1 to 0.3 mg IV immediately prior to the study, if desired.

2. At the time of the initial **LPO** ⊗ film (step 7), check that all visible margins of the stomach are well coated with barium. If not, recoat by turning **AP** ⊕ **(SUPINE)**; **RIGHT LATERAL** ⊕; **AP** ⊕ **(SUPINE)**; **LEFT LATERAL** ⊕; **LPO** ⊗. This should adequately recoat the bulb without flooding the duodenum and proximal small bowel.

3. If at step 13 **(LPO** ⊗ BULB), there is excess barium filling the duodenal bulb, three maneuvers may be used alone or in combination to better obtain an air-filled, well-coated but otherwise empty bulb.
   A. First, the patient may be turned into a steeper **LPO** ⊗ or a **LEFT LATERAL** ⊕ to allow drainage of barium retrograde into the antrum. The patient is subsequently repositioned in the **LPO** ⊗ to obtain the usual spot films.
   B. Second, the patient may be placed in the **AP** ⊕ **(SUPINE)** position. This allows barium to flow antegrade

from the bulb into the more dependent and posterior descending duodenum. The patient is then repositioned in the **LPO** ⊗ for spotting the bulb.

C. Third, the patient can be kept in the **LPO** ⊗ position and the head of the table raised to allow emptying of the bulb through the pylorus or pooling of the barium in the inferior fornix or base of the bulb with good visualization of the remainder.

4. If the duodenal bulb is directed posteriorly and cannot be properly visualized without overlapping, follow the instructions for the *Posterior Bulb Maneuver,* pages 83–85.

Chapter 4

STOMACH–SPECIAL

SALVAGING THE FAILED DOUBLE CONTRAST STUDY

POSTERIOR BULB MANEUVER

OUTLET OBSTRUCTION

PERFORATION

BILLROTH II—SINGLE CONTRAST

BILLROTH II—DOUBLE CONTRAST

GASTROSTOMY TUBE

GASTROJEJUNOSTOMY WITHOUT RESECTION
SINGLE CONTRAST

GASTROJEJUNOSTOMY WITHOUT RESECTION
DOUBLE CONTRAST

GASTRIC STAPLING

SALVAGING THE FAILED DOUBLE CONTRAST UPPER GI SERIES

1. The reasons for a failed double contrast upper GI series are myriad. However, the causes can be divided into two basic groups:
   A. Failure to maintain adequate distention, and
   B. Failure to obtain adequate coating.

   Each of these will be addressed separately.

2. Failure to maintain adequate distention can happen because the patient did not receive or ingest adequate amounts of the gas-forming granules. If the patient is not cooperative enough, or was unable to fully ingest the granules with the small amount of water provided (which may occur in patients with dysphagia or odynophagia), switch to a single contrast study immediately. Not giving additional high-density barium will permit an adequate single contrast study to be performed once normal motor function returns (after the glucagon wears off).

   If the patient was unable to maintain gaseous distention of the stomach, various reasons must be considered. Sometimes the patient is unable or unwilling to fully retain the released carbon dioxide. If the patient has a lax lower esophageal sphincter or is just otherwise unable to fully cooperate, immediately convert to a single contrast study. An additional dose of gas-forming granules and water may be administered if the examiner feels the patient would be able to cooperate fully on a second try. Additional attempts are usually futile, and also entail the administration of so much additional water to swallow the granules that the mucosal coating will then suffer. If the patient has unexpectedly large amounts of retained gastric secretions, their volume and the volume of the released carbon dioxide may just be too much for the stomach to retain. In these cases, converting to a single contrast study should be performed, but the contrast used should be somewhat denser than normal for a single contrast study so that the resultant dilution by the retained secretions does not interfere with an adequate study.

3. Failure to obtain adequate coating may also have many causes. The first one is failure to deliver the barium to the mucosal surface of interest just prior to obtaining the spot film of that area. This may be remedied by adherence to the protocol outlined in the appropriate chapter. A second reason is the presence of retained fluid interfering with the proper coating. Sometimes, additional turning of the patient, again as outlined in that chapter, may correct this problem. If the amount of retained fluid is so excessive that these measures are unsuccessful, the examination should be converted to a single contrast study.

If the double contrast exam must be converted to single contrast, and if the entire contents of a unit dose cup of high-density barium have already been administered, this will interfere with a routine single contrast study. Therefore, very-low-density barium should be used for the study of the stomach and low-density barium for the esophagus. Using low-density barium for the entire study might still result in too dense a barium to successfully penetrate, even with good external compression. Therefore, the sequence for converting a double contrast upper GI to a single one in these circumstances should be: First do the stomach and duodenal bulb and sweep with very-low-density barium and then complete the esophagus with low-density barium.

POSTERIOR DUODENAL BULB MANEUVER

If, in the performance of the double contrast UGI (at step 13, the **LPO** ⊗ of the duodenal bulb), there is a posterior duodenal bulb that cannot be adequately visualized, the following maneuvers should be performed.

1. Turn the patient into the **RIGHT LATERAL** ⊕ to recoat the duodenal bulb with barium.

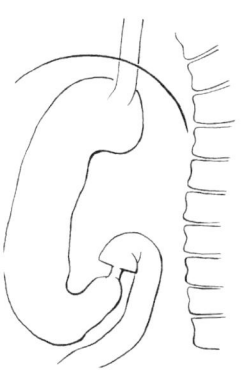

2. Turn the patient **AP** ⊕ **(SUPINE)** and then **LEFT LATERAL** ⊕.

3. Slowly "overrotate" the patient into the **LAO** ⊗ to bring the duodenal bulb off the anterior wall of the stomach. Spot the air-filled pylorus and bulb, if possible.

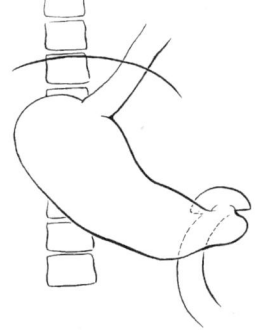

4. Raise the head of the table 75 to 80 degrees from the horizontal (almost vertical). The barium will flow along the greater curvature, stretching it out inferiorly. This converts a transverse stomach to a more longitudinally oriented one.

5. Try again to spot the bulb in the **LAO** ⊗ as air rises into it.

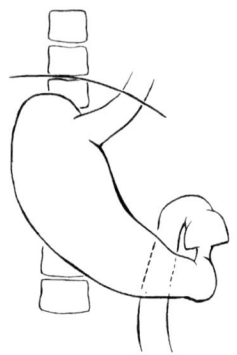

6. With the table still almost upright, turn the patient into the **LEFT LATERAL** ⊕. Then slowly turn the patient into the **LPO** ⊗ to see the bulb and sweep optimally air-filled. Spot if well visualized.

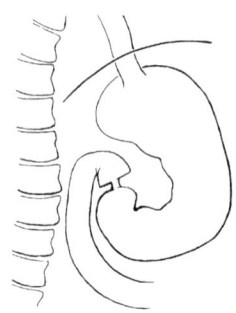

7. Holding the patient in the proper obliquity determined in step 6, lower the table toward the horizontal. Spot the bulb and sweep at whatever table angulation permits good visualization.

NOTES

1. A posterior duodenal bulb is encountered more frequently in double contrast UGI series because the rapid distention causes the stomach to dilate between two points of fixation (the GE junction and the apex of the bulb). The purpose of the above maneuvers is to stretch the stomach longitudinally between the two points, rather than transversely.

2. If on the initial **LPO** ⊗ the bulb is well-coated, start at step 3.

3. The above maneuvers must be performed rapidly before the barium coating degrades. If at any step good coating is lost, stop and restart at step 1.

4. If all steps fail, stop! Let the stomach partially empty and then retry with the residual air and barium. This sometimes works because the decreased distention lessens the severity of the transverse position of the stomach.

5. If, even with waiting, good air contrast spots of the duodenal bulb are not obtainable, have the patient drink dilute single contrast barium and spot the duodenal bulb in the **RAO** ⊗ with adequate compression. Then, turn the patient into the **LPO** ⊗ and attempt air-distended bulb shots as in the single contrast protocol.

OUTLET OBSTRUCTION

PRELIMINARY FILM: **AP ⊕ (SUPINE)** ABDOMEN

CONTRAST: MEDIUM-DENSITY BARIUM (if large amounts of retained fluid)

LOW-DENSITY BARIUM (if no fluid residua)

OVERHEADS: **AP ⊕ (SUPINE), RIGHT LATERAL ⊕**
(if complete obstruction and/or acute abdomen)

Complete single contrast routine UGI, if possible.

1. An NG tube should be in place and the stomach decompressed, if at all possible prior to the exam. More than 24 hours of decompression are recommended to allow a return of gastric tone and motility.

2. With the table horizontal, place the patient in the **RIGHT LATERAL ⊕**. Introduce a small amount (10 to 20 cc) of diluted contrast and check for retained fluid. Continue with the diluted barium if only minimal amounts are encountered. Spot the distal antrum, bulb, and sweep in overlapping segments.

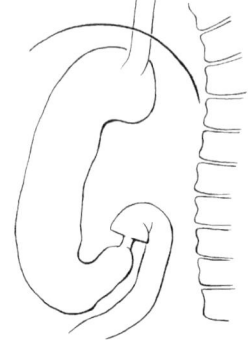

3. If no outlet obstruction is encountered, proceed as per the routine single contrast UGI.

4. If a high-grade partial or complete obstruction is noted, fluoroscope intermittently in the **RIGHT LATERAL** ⊕ to check for filling of the bulb and sweep.

5. Turn the patient **AP** ⊕ **(SUPINE)** and spot the distal antrum and the bulb and sweep, if opacified.

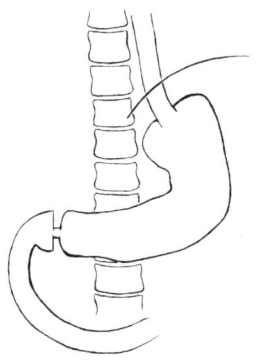

6. Turn the patient into the **LPO** ⊗. Spot the air-filled distal half of the stomach and the bulb and sweep, if possible. The NG tube may be used to introduce the air, if necessary.

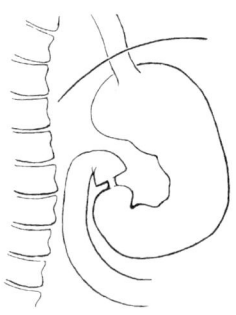

7. If an obstruction is seen, use the NG tube to drain the stomach of residual barium, fluid, and debris prior to the patient's return to the floor, to prevent possible aspiration.

UPPER GI FOR PERFORATED VISCUS

PRELIMINARY FILMS: **AP ⊕ (SUPINE)** ABDOMEN

AP ⊕ (UPRIGHT) ABDOMEN TO INCLUDE DIAPHRAGMS

OR

LEFT LATERAL ⊕ DECUBITUS

CONTRAST: WATER SOLUBLE CONTRAST

OVERHEADS: **AP ⊕ (SUPINE), RIGHT LATERAL ⊕, LEFT LATERAL ⊕**

IF POSSIBLE: **PA ⊖ (PRONE), RAO ⊗**

1. With the table horizontal, start with the patient in the **RIGHT LATERAL ⊕** position. Have the patient swallow one small mouthful of contrast. Follow the bolus to the GE junction and spot this area.

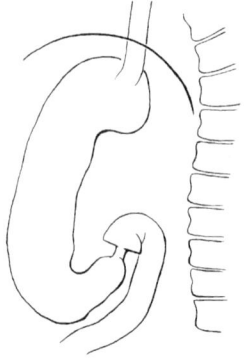

2. Continue to slowly fill the stomach with contrast. Stop at the first sign of extravasation. Spot the area of leakage.

3. If no extravasation, continue to fill the distal stomach, bulb, and sweep, and spot these areas in overlapping segments.

4. Turn the patient **AP** ⊕ **(SUPINE)** and spot the distal antrum, bulb, and sweep again.

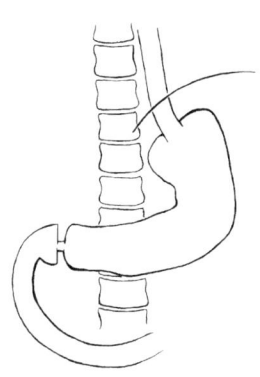

5. Return the patient to the **RIGHT LATERAL** ⊕ and keep the patient in this position for 5 to 10 min. before obtaining the overheads.

NOTES

1. Prone and prone oblique films may not be feasible, no matter how desirable, in a patient with an acute abdomen, abdominal pain, and/or tenderness. Therefore, the anterior wall of the stomach and duodenal bulb are not well examined using this technique (see below).

2. If no extravasation is seen even after the delayed overheads, the exam should be continued with medium-density barium since many perforations can be missed on water soluble studies.

3. Compression should be used sparingly, since pressure on previously diseased bowel may cause it to rupture.

BILLROTH II–SINGLE CONTRAST

PRELIMINARY FILM: **AP ⊕ (SUPINE)** ABDOMEN

CONTRAST: LOW-DENSITY BARIUM

OVERHEADS: **AP ⊕ (SUPINE), PA ⊖ (PRONE), RIGHT LATERAL ⊕, RPO ⊗, LAO ⊗** ABDOMEN

1. With the table horizontal, start with the patient in the **RAO ⊗**. Have the patient swallow a small bolus of barium.

2. Turn the patient **PA ⊖ (PRONE)**. Place the compression paddle under the patient and spot the gastric pouch and gastrojejunostomy in mucosal relief as it projects to the right of the spine.

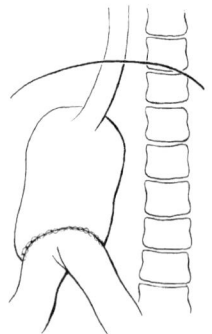

3. Turn the patient **LAO ⊗** and again spot the gastric pouch and anastamosis in mucosal relief as they project just to the right or over the spine. The undersurface of the jejunal side of the anastamosis should be "open" without overlapping of the afferent and efferent limbs.

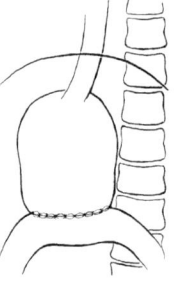

STOMACH—SPECIAL

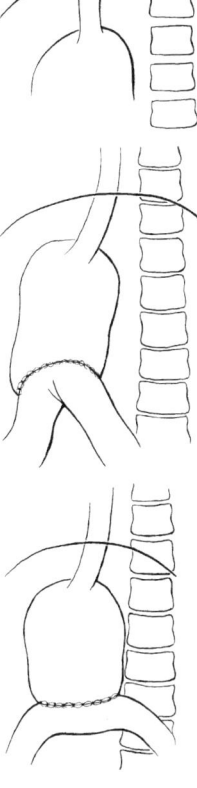

4. Return the patient to the **RAO** ⊗ position and have the patient rapidly drink barium to distend the esophagus. Spot the esophagus in overlapping segments as it projects to the right of the spine. Have the patient perform a Valsalva maneuver and spot the GE junction for a possible hiatal hernia.

5. Turn the patient **PA** ⊕ **(PRONE)** and spot the fully-distended gastric pouch and anastamosis with compression.

6. Turn the patient **LAO** ⊗ and re-spot, as in step 5 above.

7. Turn the patient **AP** ⊕ **(SU-PINE)** and spot the gastric remnant and the anastomosis as they project to the left of the spine.

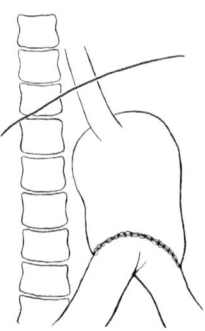

8. Turn the patient **RPO** ⊘ and spot the stomach and anastomosis as they overlie the spine.

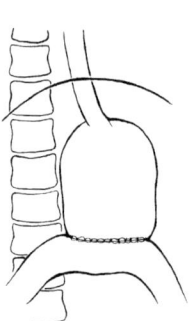

NOTES

1. 0.3 mg of glucagon may be administered intravenously if rapid emptying is expected or encountered.

2. Semi-upright tilting of the table may sometimes be of help in seeing and evaluating the gastrojejunal anastomosis.

3. Be very careful not to overfill the gastric pouch. If any doubt exists as to its emptying, postpone the esophageal component of the exam until a satisfactory gastric pouch exam is completed.

BILLROTH II–DOUBLE CONTRAST

PRELIMINARY FILM: **AP ⊕ (SUPINE)** ABDOMEN

CONTRAST: HIGH-DENSITY BARIUM
LOW-DENSITY BARIUM

OVERHEADS: **PA ⊕ (PRONE)**

1. Administer 0.3 mg of glucagon intravenously.

2. Start with the patient in the **RAO** ⊗ position and the table horizontal. Have the patient swallow a small bolus of contrast. Spot the esophagus in mucosal relief in overlapping segments as it projects to the right of the spine.

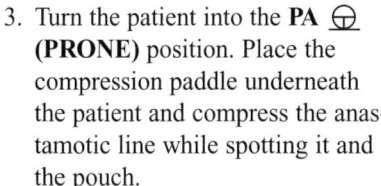

3. Turn the patient into the **PA ⊕ (PRONE)** position. Place the compression paddle underneath the patient and compress the anastamotic line while spotting it and the pouch.

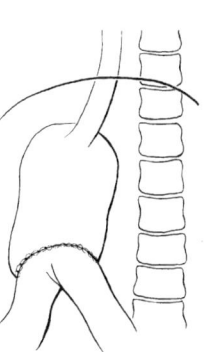

4. Turn the patient **LAO** ⊗ and obtain a compression spot of the gastric pouch and anastamosis. In this position the anastamosis should be "open" without overlapping along its inferior border.

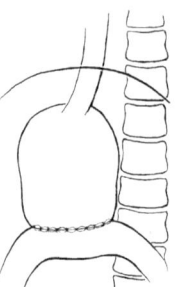

5. Raise the table to the full upright position. Start with the patient in the **LPO** ⊗ position. Administer the gas-forming crystals with 10 to 15 cc of water. Have the patient rapidly swallow half a cup of the high-density barium (60 to 70 cc) while spotting the air-filled esophagus in overlapping segments as it projects just to the left of the spine.

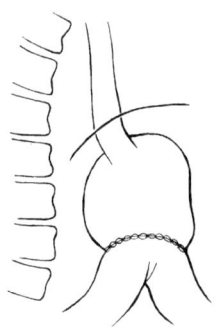

6. Turn the patient into the **AP** ⊕ **(SUPINE)** position and lower the table to the horizontal plane. Because the anastamosis is usually along the anterior wall of the stomach, the **AP** ⊕ **(SUPINE)** position is the best in which to lower the patient and prevent premature emptying of the stomach.

7. Turn the patient from the **AP** ⊕ **(SUPINE)** to **LEFT LATERAL** ⊕ to **PA** ⊕ **(PRONE)** to **LEFT LATERAL** ⊕ to **AP**

⊕ (**SUPINE**). These turns avoid placing the right side in a dependent position, allowing more rapid emptying.

8. Spot the well-coated and air-filled gastric remnant and anastamosis in the **AP** ⊕ (**SUPINE**) position. It should project to the left of the spine.

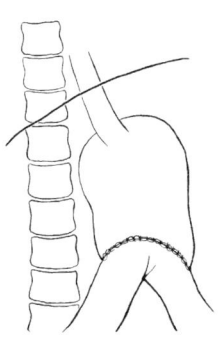

9. Turn the patient into a minimal **RPO** ⊘ and spot as above. Part of the pouch or anastomosis may project over the spine.

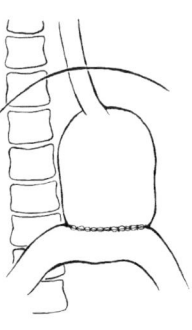

10. Steepen the obliquity **RPO** (⊘) and spot again, as above. In this position a more significant portion of the pouch projects over the spine.

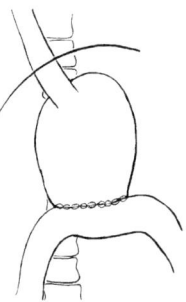

11. Turn the patient into the **RIGHT LATERAL** ⊕. Spot the air-filled gastric pouch and the barium-filled gastrojejunostomy.

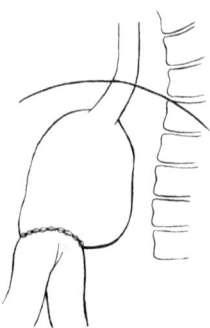

12. Turn the patient into the **PA** ⊖ **(PRONE)** position and spot the air-filled pouch as it projects to the right of the spine.

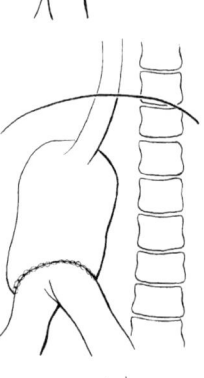

13. Turn the patient **LAO** ⊗ and spot the pouch and anastamosis as it crosses over the spine.

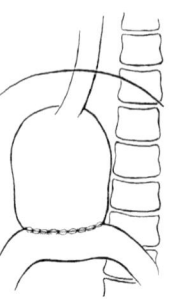

14. Turn the patient into the **RAO** ⊗. Have the patient rapidly drink the low-density barium. Spot the esophagus in overlapping segments. Have the patient perform a Valsalva maneuver and spot the GE junction for a possible hiatal hernia.

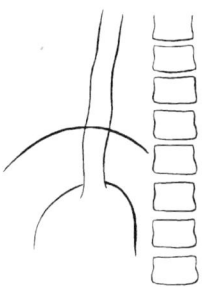

NOTES

1. Always start with a small bolus of barium. Large amounts of contrast may overfill the gastric pouch, obscuring the anastamotic site. Once this happens it is very difficult to properly evaluate this area.

2. If the gastric pouch overdistends with air and overhangs the anastamosis, obtain the spot films in the semi-erect position. Gravity will help pull the ananstamotic area inferiorly, while the gastric pouch will remain relatively fixed in position. This will usually enable better visualization.

GASTROSTOMY TUBE

PRELIMINARY FILM: **AP ⊕ (SUPINE) ABDOMEN**

CONTRAST: WATER SOLUBLE (if checking tube position or leakage)

LOW-DENSITY BARIUM (if checking for reflux or gastroduodenal pathology)

OVERHEADS: **AP ⊕ (SUPINE), RIGHT LATERAL ⊕**

1. Start with the patient **AP ⊕ (SUPINE)** and the table horizontal. Hand inject a small amount of contrast. Check fluoroscopically for any extravasation of contrast.

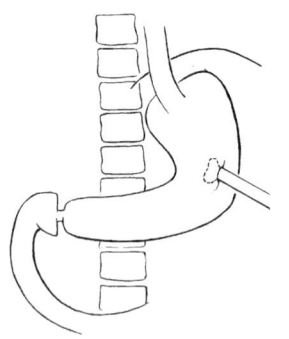

2. If none is observed, turn the patient into the **RIGHT LATERAL ⊕** and check again. If any leakage is observed, spot the area immediately and stop the exam. If no leakage is seen, proceed as below.

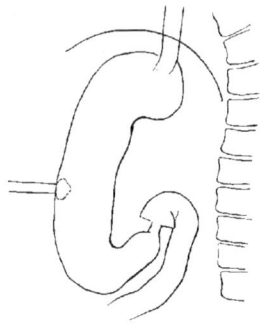

STOMACH—SPECIAL

3. Proceed with the patient in the **RIGHT LATERAL** ⊕ position. Continue to hand inject barium in 20 cc increments to outline the distal antrum, duodenal bulb, and sweep. Spot these areas as they become barium-filled and distended.

4. Turn the patient **AP** ⊕ **(SUPINE)** and spot the distal antrum and sweep. The barium-filled fundus may also be spotted at this time.

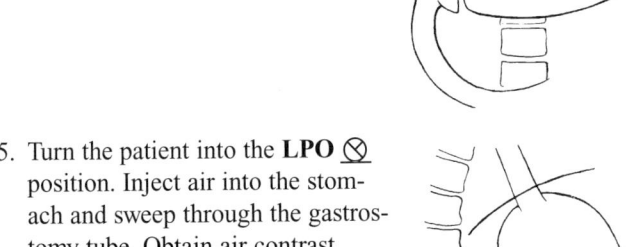

5. Turn the patient into the **LPO** ⊗ position. Inject air into the stomach and sweep through the gastrostomy tube. Obtain air contrast views of the distal antrum and bulb.

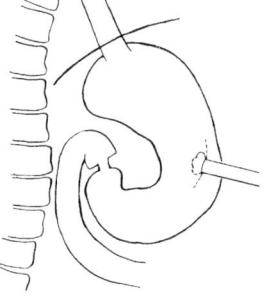

BYPASS GASTROJEJUNOSTOMY WITHOUT RESECTION

PRELIMINARY FILM: **AP** ⊕ **(SUPINE)** ABDOMEN

CONTRAST: LOW-DENSITY BARIUM

OVERHEADS: **AP** ⊕ **(SUPINE), RAO** ⊗**, RIGHT LATERAL** ⊕**, RPO,** ⊗**, LPO** ⊗ OF STOMACH, **PA** ⊕ **(PRONE)** FULL ABDOMEN

1. Place the table level and the patient in an **RAO** ⊗ projection. Have the patient swallow a small bolus of barium and follow this fluoroscopically to the stomach. Spot, in overlapping segments, the collapsed, mucosal relief of the coated esophagus. The esophaus should project to the right of the spine, on the same side as the stomach.

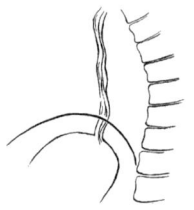

2. With the small amount of barium coating the gastric rugae, place a compression paddle underneath the patient and inflate the balloon to apply sufficient pressure to spread apart the folds and "see through" the barium. Spot the body (A) and antrum (B). Spot the duodenal bulb (C) and sweep (D), if they fill. The bulb should not be superimposed upon the spine al-

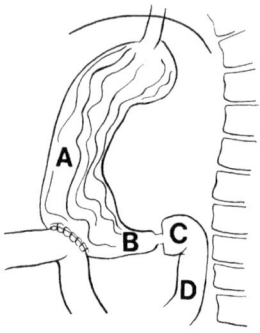

3. Turn the patient into the **LAO** ⊗ position and compress the proximal greater curvature of the antrum (the usual surgical site).

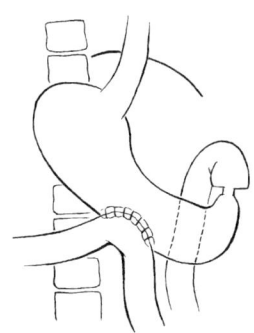

4. Return the patient to the **RAO** ⊗ position. Have the patient rapidly drink large amounts of barium. Spot the fully distended esophagus in overlapping segments. Have the patient strain (Valsalva maneuver) while the esophagus is fully distended just prior to spotting the gastroesophageal junction.

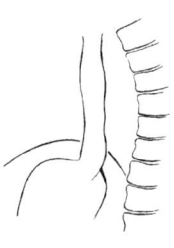

5. Using the previously placed compression paddle, spot the fully-distended stomach and duodenum with adequate compression to see fold detail through the barium. Move the paddle to fully examine both the body (A) and antrum (B), as well as the bulb (C) and sweep (D) if they fill.

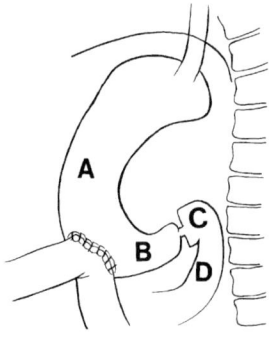

6. Remove the compression paddle. Turn the patient into the **RIGHT LATERAL** ⊕. Spot the distal antrum and barium-filled bypass loop.

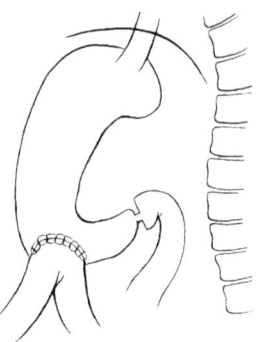

7. Continue turning the patient into the **RPO** ⊘. Spot the mid-portion of the stomach, with particular attention to the lesser curvature. If the barium is too dense to see detail in the stomach, use the compression paddle on the anterior abdominal wall to aid in penetration. The mid-portion of the lesser curvature should be superimposed over the spine or just to the right of it.

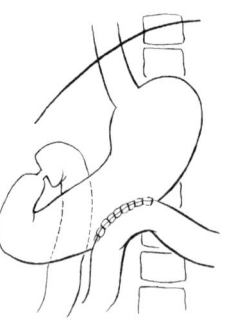

8. Apply compression, as needed, to see the anastamosis "en face" along the greater curvature, with the patient still in the **RPO** ⊘.

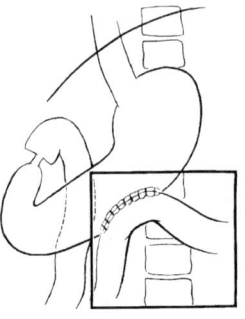

9. With barium covering the GE junction, while still in the **RPO** ⊘, have the patient strain (Valsalva) and watch to see if barium refluxes into the distal esophagus. Spot the superior extent of the reflux and make note of how promptly the refluxed material is cleared from the entire esophagus.

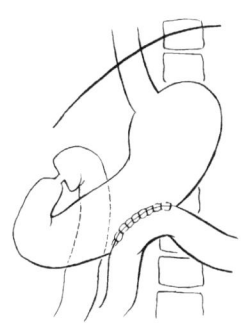

10. Turn the patient into the **AP** ⊕ **(SUPINE)** position. Spot the midportion of the stomach, which should be partially air-filled. The antrum will be superimposed over the spine, while the bulb and descending duodenum, if opacified, will be on the right, away from the stomach.

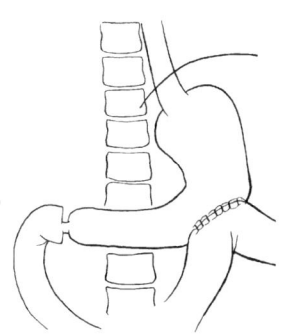

11. Turn the patient into the **LPO** ⊘ position and allow air to rise into the distal antrum and, possibly, the duodenal bulb. Spot the air-distended and well-coated antrum (A). If filled, spot the bulb (B) and sweep (C).

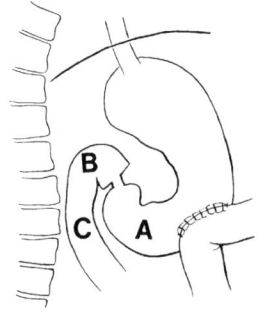

NOTE

Pay particular attention during fluoroscopy as to whether the duodenum fills antegrade through the pylorus or retrograde through the gastrojejunostomy.

GASTROJEJUNOSTOMY WITHOUT RESECTION–DOUBLE CONTRAST

PRELIMINARY FILM: **AP ⊕ (SUPINE)** ABDOMEN

CONTRAST: HIGH-DENSITY BARIUM
LOW-DENSITY BARIUM

OVERHEADS: **PA ⊕ (PRONE)** ABDOMEN

1. Administer glucagon 0.3 mg IV to slow gastric emptying.

2. Start with the table horizontal and the patient in the **RAO** ⊗ position. Have the patient swallow a small bolus of the high-density barium. Spot the collapsed, coated mucosal relief of the esophagus in overlapping segments. The esophagus should project to the right of the spine, on the same side as the stomach.

3. Place the compression paddle under the patient. Apply sufficient compression to "see through" the barium and visualize the rugal folds. Spot the gastric body (A) and antrum (B), as well as the duodenal bulb (C) and sweep (D), if they fill.

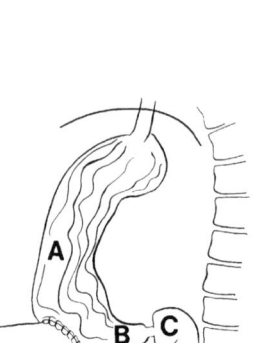

4. Turn the patient into the **LAO** ⊘ and take a compression spot (mucosal relief) of the proximal antrum to view the anastamosis "en face."

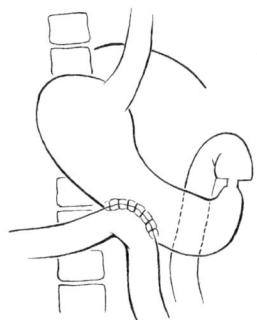

5. Turn the patient **AP** ⊕ **(SUPINE)** and bring the table to the full upright position.

6. Place the patient **LPO** ⊘. Have the patient swallow the gas-producing granules with 10 to 15 cc of water. Immediately follow the granules with very rapid gulping of the high-density barium. As the esophagus becomes air-filled and distended, take overlapping spot films of the well-coated esophagus as it projects to the left of the spine, on the same side as the stomach.

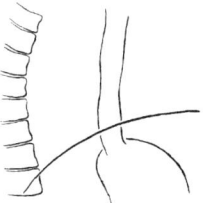

7. Turn the patient **PA** ⊕ **(PRONE)**, facing the table top and lower the table to the horizontal plane.

8. Turn the patient quickly in the following sequence: **PA** ⊕ **(PRONE)**; **LEFT LATERAL** ⊕; **AP** ⊕ **(SUPINE)**; **LEFT**

**LATERAL ⊕; PA ⊖
(PRONE); LEFT LATERAL
⊕; AP ⊕ (SUPINE); RIGHT
LATERAL ⊕; PA ⊖
(PRONE); LEFT LATERAL
⊕**; ending in the **LPO ⊗**.

9. In the **LPO ⊗** position, spot the distal half of the stomach, which is air-filled and well-coated. The entire stomach should project to the left of the spine.

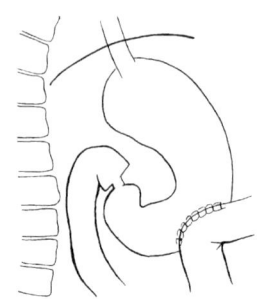

10. Turn the patient **AP ⊕ (SUPINE)**. Spot the distal half of the air-filled, well-coated stomach. The distal portion of the antrum should overlie the spine.

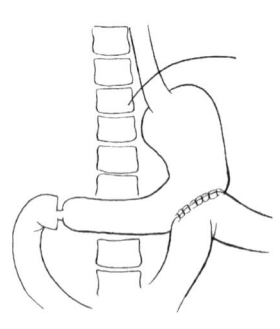

11. Turn the patient into a shallow **RPO ⊘**. Spot the distal half of the lesser curvature as it projects just to the right of the spine. The gastrojejunal anastamosis may be seen "en face" just over the spine or minimally off to either side.

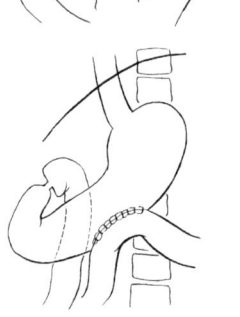

STOMACH—SPECIAL 107

12. Turn the patient into the **RIGHT LATERAL** ⊕ position. Spot the air-filled fundus and proximal body of the stomach. They should project anterior to the spine.

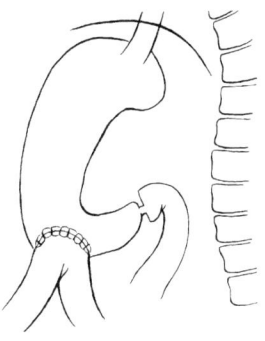

13. Turn the patient into the **LPO** ⊗. Spot the air-filled distal antrum (A) and bulb (B) and sweep (C), if opacified. They should project to the left of the spine on the same side as the stomach.

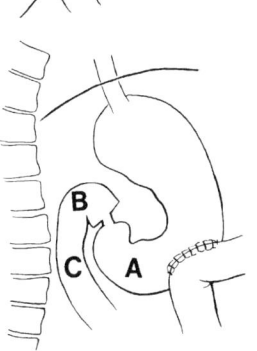

14. Turn the patient into the **RAO** ⊗ position. Have the patient rapidly drink the dilute barium to fully distend the esophagus. Spot the distended esophagus in overlapping segments; it should project to the right of the spine. Spot the GE junction immediately, following a Valsalva maneuver, performed while the esophagus is still barium-filled.

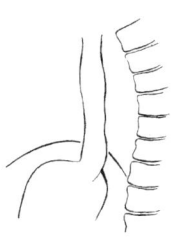

NOTE

1. Pay particular attention during fluoroscopy to whether the duodenum fills antegrade through the pylorus or retrograde through the gastrojejunostomy.

GASTRIC STAPLING

There are too many variations of gastric stapling procedures to be reviewed in a book of this size; therefore, the following general principles are recommended:

1. As always, try to communicate with the surgeon before studying the patient.

2. If a gastric resection or exclusion was performed, then a variant of the gastrojejunostomy bypass without resection protocol may be of value, keeping in mind the smaller volume of the stomach remnant.

3. If a Mason's vertical banded gastroplasty was performed, then only small amounts of barium should be used since the gastric resevoir only holds approximately 30 cc. The **RPO** ⊘ position should be used to examine the staple line that separates the pouch from the remainder of the stomach.

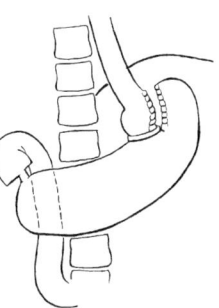

Chapter 5

SMALL BOWEL–ROUTINE

DEDICATED SMALL BOWEL STUDY
ENTEROCLYSIS TUBE PLACEMENT
ENTEROCLYSIS—SINGLE CONTRAST
ENTEROCYLSIS—DOUBLE CONTRAST

DEDICATED SMALL BOWEL STUDY

PRELIMINARY FILM: AP ⊕ **(SUPINE)** ABDOMEN

CONTRAST: LOW-DENSITY BARIUM

OVERHEADS: **PA** ⊕ **(PRONE)**, **PA** ⊕ ABDOMEN (with 30 degrees caudal angulation)

1. Start by administering 360 cc of barium p.o.

2. Take an immediate overhead film after the patient has finished drinking. Fluoroscope all visualized loops utilizing manual compression with a paddle. Spot any abnormality.

3. Continue with intermittent filming and fluoroscopy at 15 to 30 min. intervals until the cecum is reached. If the stomach is empty on any overhead film or during fluoroscopic evaluation, administer another 360 cc of barium.

4. When the cecum is reached and all proximal loops are filled with barium, spot the entire small bowel using compression as follows:

   A. The jejunal loops in the LUQ are generally seen best without overlap in the moderate **RPO** ⊘.

   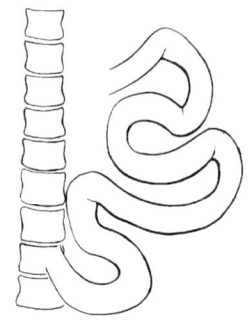

   B. The distal jejunal loops in the LLQ are best seen without overlap in a less steep **RPO** ⊘.

   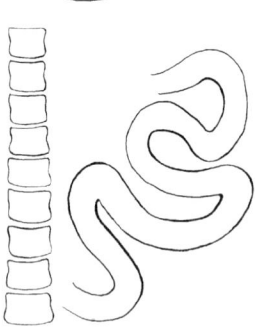

   C. The mid-ileal loops very often lie in the RUQ just inferior to the hepatic flexure and are best visualized in a minimal **LPO** ⊘ (similar to spotting the hepatic flexure).

   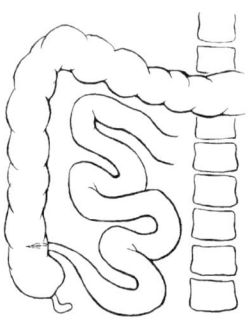

D. The pelvic loops of ileum are the most difficult to fully visualize. If the **AP ⊕ (SUPINE)** and both supine obliques **(RPO ⊘, LPO ⊗)** fail to adequately visualize this segment, the patient should be turned into the **PA ⊕ (PRONE)** position. The head of the table should be lowered 15 to 20 degrees and the compression paddle placed under the patient in the suprapubic region. It should then be inflated forcing the loops out of the deep pelvic recesses.

E. The ileocecal valve and the terminal ileum are best seen in a minimal degree of **RPO ⊘**. This is because the valve in usually posterior in location and the **RPO ⊘** allows it to be seen "en face."

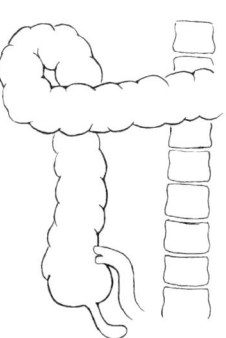

NOTES

1. If the terminal ileum and/or the cecum cannot be readily isolated, then the patient should be turned into the **LPO ⊗** position. This should allow the examiner to see the hepatic flexure. The colon should be traced backwards with fluoroscopy until the cecum is seen. Once this area is identified, the proper spot films of the terminal ileum can be obtained.

2. If still unsucessful in localizing the terminal ileum and cecum, the patient may be turned **LEFT LATERAL** ⊕ and kept in that position for a few minutes. This allows air in the distal half of the colon to rise into the right colon, aiding in visualizing the cecum.

3. If the maneuver outlined in note 2 is not successful, then a peroral pneumocolon (as described on pages 133–134.) should be performed.

4. Another way of displacing the ileal loops out of the pelvis is to insufflate air into the rectum, as in the performance of a peroral pneumocolon. Instead of instilling sufficient air to fill the entire colon and reflux into the small bowel, only enough air is used to cause the sigmoid colon to fill while displacing the dependent and barium-filled loops of small bowel.

ENTEROCLYSIS TUBE PLACEMENT

MATERIALS: MAGLINTE ENTEROCLYSIS CATHETER (COOK INC.)

    OR

    E-Z-EM ENTEROCLYSIS CATHETER

    2% LIDOCAINE JELLY

1. Start with the patient in the **AP ⊕ (SUPINE)** position. Ascertain which nostril is the more patent by alternately occluding one side with finger pressure and having the patient sniff through the other.

2. Using the more patent nostril, introduce the lidocaine by placing the gel at the orifice and having the patient sniff. As a general rule, anesthetizing the oropharynx should be avoided to prevent interference with the normal swallowing mechanism (and allowing tracheal rather than esophageal placement).

3. Introduce the catheter without the stiffening wire in place. This allows the floppy unsupported catheter to easily negotiate the right angle turn at the posterior nasopharynx. The catheter should be guided directly posterior into the nose, perpendicular to the frontal

plane of the skull, rather than parallel to the bridge of the nose towards the orbit. The right-angle bend noted above is most easily negotiated with the neck in a neutral position. Flexion helps close off the nasopharynx and makes it difficult to make the turn. Extension makes inadvertant tracheal placement more likely. Continue to advance the catheter until the patient feels like gagging. At that point, withdraw the catheter 1 to 2 cm and allow the patient to catch his breath.

4. Have the patient flex his neck, with the chin almost touching the chest. Have the patient swallow his own saliva three times in rapid succession. Rapidly, but gently, advance the catheter with the second and third, but not the first swallow. Not using the first swallow allows you to judge the patient's swallowing ability, as well as adjust your timing for the catheter advancement.

5. If the patient is still able to talk at this time, the catheter is most likely in the esophagus. Confirm this with fluoroscopy. The catheter should "split the carina," continuing past it in the midline.

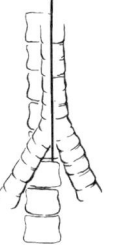

6. Continue to advance the tube until it enters the stomach. If the tube is bent back upon itself in the esophagus, one may attempt a "double back" maneuver, as explained below. However, I prefer to continue advancing the tube until it passes the GE junction, where it will uncoil itself in the larger gastric lumen.

7. When in the stomach, the guide wire should be inserted. If there are two ends to the wire (a straight and a "hockey stick"), the angled "hockey stick" should be used. This allows some torque control and steerability. The tip should be directed towards the lesser curvature and the tube/wire combination advanced into the antrum.

A. If the guide wire has only a straight end or if the antrum cannot be easily reached (for example, if it coils in the fundus), the patient should be placed in the **RIGHT LATERAL** ⊕ position. The catheter/wire combination should be advanced so it proceeds anteriorly (away from the spine) into the antrum.

B. If the patient cannot be turned, or if steps 7 and 7A are unsuccesful, then a "double back" maneuver should be performed with the patient in the **AP** ⊕ **(SUPINE)** position. As the catheter and wire coil in the fundus (A), they should be further inserted so that the catheter "buckles" down into the body (B). The wire should be withdrawn until it is at the apex of the buckle (∗). Then, simultaneously and at the same rate, the straight end of the wire is advanced as the catheter is withdrawn. If this is done properly, the net effect is to shorten the catheter while the position of the wire's tip and the apex of the bend remain unchanged (C). Ultimately, the end of the catheter is located at or distal to the in-

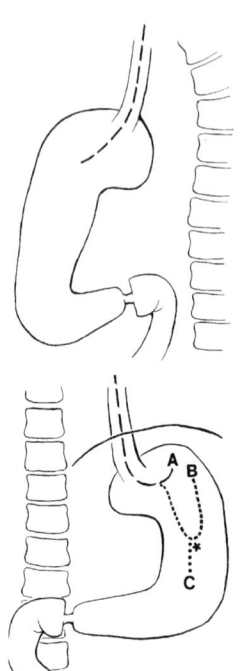

cisura, allowing easy advancement into the antrum.

8. The wire in now placed 2 to 3 cm short of the catheter tip, leaving a short segment of catheter unsupported by the wire. This soft, floppy tip is essential in not traumatizing the pylorus and inducing pylorospasm. The straight end of the wire is best used in traversing the sphincter. The catheter/wire combination usually lies parallel to and along the greater curvature of the stomach. The bent "hockey stick" end will cause the catheter tip to lie perpendicular to the pyloric channel, rather than parallel to it.

9. At this time the patient should be placed in a fairly steep **LPO** ⊗. This allows air to rise into the distal antrum and outline the pylorus and duodenal bulb. In a sense the bulb may be thought to fall over the outstretched catheter/wire, rather than the latter being pushed through the opening.

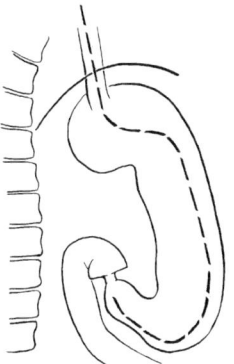

10. As the catheter/wire is advanced, it should be monitored as to its curvature. If it bends anteriorly, away from the spine (A), it probably is doubling back upon itself in the antrum. If it goes superiorly, parallel to and then posteriorly toward the spine (B), it probably is in the duodenal bulb. Withdrawal of the wire and injection of 50 to 60 cc of air will confirm the position or help outline the correct route of placement.

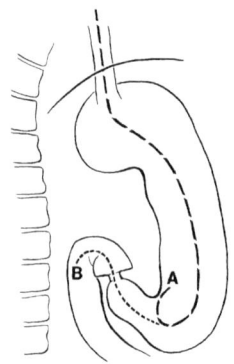

11. Once the catheter/wire is past the bulb, the patient should be returned to the **AP ⊕ (SUPINE)** position. The catheter should be stripped off the wire and advanced to just past the spine, in the third portion of the duodenum (for bleeding cases) or to the ligament of Treitz (in all other cases). This is accomplished by alternately advancing the catheter and withdrawing the wire 2 to 3 cm at a time. Care should be taken to prevent the wire from passing beyond the bulb, because the stiff wire is difficult to bend around the acute angles of the thin-walled duodenum.

12. If the catheter starts to bend back upon itself, one should withdraw

it slightly and then re-advance it. This usually will allow the catheter to seek the right path.

13. The balloon should be inflated under fluoroscopic observation with 10 to 15 cc of air. If the borders of the balloon appear abnormally flattened, then the balloon is overinflated in relation to the bowel diameter and should be partially decompressed.

NOTE

Many authors advocate the usage of Reglan (metaclopramide) to aid in the passage of the catheter; 5 to 10 mg, either p.o. or IV, can be used to enhance gastric peristalsis and relax the pyloric sphincter. Some authors also advocate the usage of Valium (diazepam) or other sedatives to help make the examination more comfortable for the patient. I have not found great utility in either medication. However, the ability to fill the entire small bowel more rapidly does provide a theoretic advantage over the use of Reglan.

ENTEROCLYSIS–SINGLE CONTRAST

PRELIMINARY FILM: **AP ⊕ (SUPINE)** ABDOMEN

CONTRAST: LOW-DENSITY BARIUM

OVERHEADS: **PA ⊕ (PRONE), AP ⊕ (SUPINE), RAO ⊗, LAO ⊗** ABDOMEN

1. Place the catheter as described previously on pages 117–123.

2. Elevate the head of the table 15 degrees. Place the patient in a mild **LPO ⊗**. Start the infusion of barium.

3. Adjust the flow rate so that the barium moves ahead through the small bowel at a steady rate without undue dilatation of the proximal jejunum. If dilatation occurs, slow the infusion rate of the pump in 5 to 10 cc/min. increments.

4. If barium flows rapidly ahead through the small bowel in a narrow, nondistended stream, increase the infusion rate in the same 5 to 10 cc/min. increments.

5. As the LLQ starts to fill, spot the LUQ well-distended loops in a moderate **RPO** ⊘ position. Use compression to separate loops and "see through" the barium.

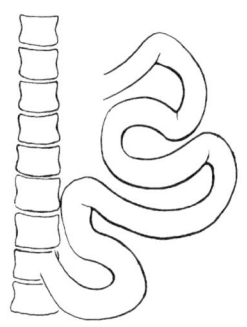

6. When the LLQ is opacified and fully distended, spot those loops in a slightly less steep **RPO** ⊘.

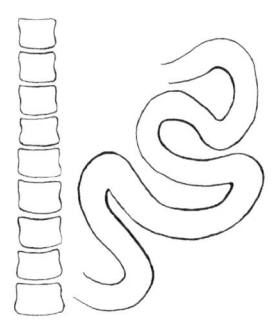

7. As the pelvic loops fill spot them in the **AP** ⊕ **(SUPINE)** position. Use both obliques **(RPO** ⊘ **, LPO** ⊗**)** if needed to further evaluate these areas. Compression of the deep pelvic loops is difficult and **PRONE** (⊖) **PA** compression with 10 to 15 degrees of Trendelenburg may be necessary as well.

8. Spot the small bowel loops just inferior to the hepatic flexure in a minimal **LPO** ⊗.

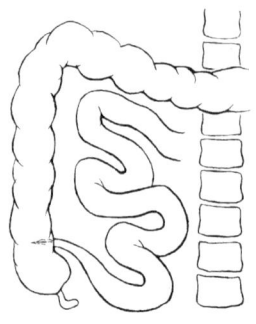

9. Spot the terminal ileum in a mild **RPO** ⊘.

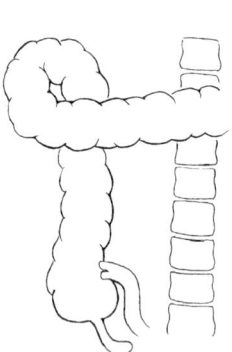

10. The pump should continue to infuse during the performance of the overheads to insure continued distention.

NOTES

1. Periodically check the duodenal sweep for reflux. If this occurs, raise the head of the table 15 degrees and place the patient in the **LPO** ⊗ position. The pump infusion rate should also be lowered 10 to 15 cc/min..

2. Alternatively, at step 10, the pump may be stopped and glucagon 1.0 mg IV administered to stop intestinal motility.

ENTEROCLYSIS–DOUBLE CONTRAST

PRELIMINARY FILM: **AP ⊕ (SUPINE)** ABDOMEN

CONTRAST: MEDIUM-DENSITY BARIUM
METHYLCELLULOSE 0.5% AQUEOUS SOLUTION

OVERHEADS: **AP ⊕ (SUPINE)**, **PA ⊕ (PRONE)**, SHALLOW **RAO** ⊗ AND **LAO** ⊗, ABDOMEN; **LATERAL** PELVIS (if necessary)

1. Place the tube as described on pages 117–123.

2. Elevate the head of the table 15 degrees and place the patient in a mild **LPO** ⊗. Start the infusion of barium.

3. Adjust the flow rate of the barium infusion pump so that the contrast moves ahead at a steady rate without undue dilatation of the jejunum. If dilatation occurs, slow the pump in 5 to 10 cc/min. increments.

4. If barium flows rapidly ahead in a narrow stream, then increase the flow rate in 5 to 10 cc/min. increments.

5. As the LLQ fills, spot the LUQ barium-distended loops in the **RPO** ⊘ projection using compression.

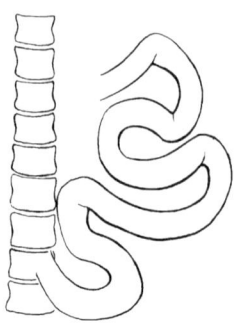

6. When the mid-pelvic loops of small bowel opacify, change the infusion from barium to methylcellulose.

7. Respot the LUQ loops as double contrast develops.

8. As double contrast develops in the LLQ, spot these in a slightly less-steep **RPO** ⊘ than needed for the LUQ.

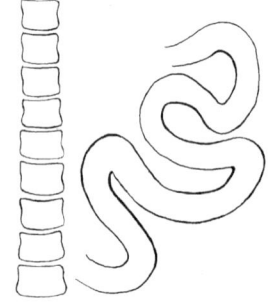

SMALL BOWEL—ROUTINE

9. As additional portions of the small bowel are seen in double contrast, spot them. The RUQ loops inferior to the hepatic flexure and the mid-abdominal loops are usually best seen in a mild **LPO ⊘**.

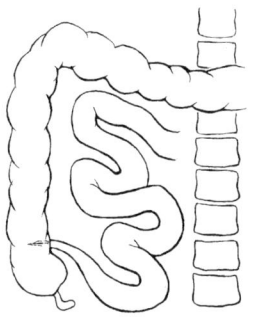

10. Spot the terminal ileum as double contrast is seen in a mild **RPO ⊘**.

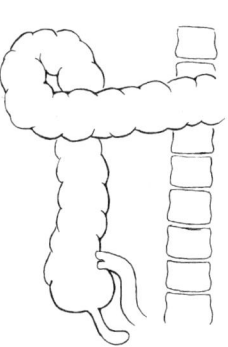

11. Keep the methylcellulose infusing during the overhead filming.

NOTES

1. Periodically check the duodenal sweep for reflux. If this occurs, raise the head of the table 15 degrees and place the patient in the **LPO ⊘** position. The pump infusion rate should also be lowered 10 to 15 cc/min.

2. Alternatively, at step 11, the pump may be stopped and glucagon 1.0 mg IV administered to stop intestinal activity.

3. Limit the use of compression and changes in patient position once the methylcellulose infusion begins. Both of these actions promote mixing of the barium and methylcellulose resulting in a dilute single contrast exam rather than the intended double contrast.

4. If the pelvic loops distend with contrast but there is no further progression in filling the more-distal small bowel, or if the methylcellulose appears to flow over and past the barium in these loops, turn the patient **PRONE (PA ⊕)**. This aids peristalsis and will permit the dense barium to flow out of the dependent pelvic loops.

5. A lateral film of the pelvis is especially helpful in women who have had a hysterectomy in the past. Subsequent to this surgery the small bowel loops have a tendency to lie in the deep pelvic recesses where they can be hard to assess.

Chapter 6

SMALL BOWEL–SPECIAL

    PERORAL PNEUMOCOLON
    OBSTRUCTION
    PERFORATION
    ILEOSTOMY
    ILEO-ANAL "J" OR "S"

PERORAL PNEUMOCOLON

Performed as an adjunct to a small bowel follow through, dedicated small bowel series, or a single contrast enteroclysis. This exams allows a double contrast view of the distal and terminal ileum.

OVERHEADS: **AP ⊕ (SUPINE), PA ⊖ (PRONE)** ABDOMEN

EQUIPMENT: SOFT RED RUBBER CATHETER OR FOLEY CATHETER

OR

BARIUM ENEMA TIP WITH ATTACHED TUBING AND AN AIR-INSUFFLATOR

1. Insert the catheter with its attached tubing and insufflator into the rectum.

2. When the cecum is opacified, air is gently insufflated with the patient in the **AP ⊕ (SUPINE)** position until the entire colon is air-filled.

3. With continued slow insufflation, air should reflux through the ileocecal valve into the terminal ileum.

4. If the valve is competent and no air refluxes, 1.0 mg of glucagon may be administered intravenously

to help relax the colonic musculature to allow reflux.

5. If reflux still does not occur, turn the patient prone. Air will rise and pass more readily through the more posteriorly located ileocecal valve.

6. If severe intestinal cramps are encountered, 25 to 50 mg of meperidine may rarely be needed to complete the exam.

7. Spot films of the small bowel loops of interest, should be obtained as indicated.

NOTE

1. If during the administration of air the patient cannot retain sufficient amounts for adequate colonic distention, place the patient in the **LEFT LATERAL** ⊕ and let the air in the transverse colon rise into the ascending colon and cecum. Very often this will deliver sufficient air to allow a succesful study of the terminal ileum.

SMALL BOWEL OBSTRUCTION

1. Proceed as per the dedicated small bowel series protocol but:

2. Observe the rate of small bowel filling between the initial film and the first delayed film. If slow flow is identified, then lengthen the time intervals between films, from 30 min. to 1 to 2 hr., until 4 to 6 hr. after the start of the procedure. At that time 4 to 5 hr. intervals are appropriate.

3. Notify the responsible nursing staff that, if the patient has an NG or nasoenteric tube in situ, it should not be used for decompression. This will prevent inadvertent removal of the contrast.

NOTES

1. Use additional overhead views to better visualize potential sites of obstruction.
   A. If an anterior abdominal wall hernia is suspected, a lateral film of the abdomen—including the anterior abdominal wall in profile—is recommended.
   B. If an incisional hernia is suspected, then an oblique that places the incision tangential to the X-ray beam should be performed.
   C. Both obliques (prone [**RAO** ⊗, **LAO** ⊗] if possible) may help in separating overlapping loops of normal or dilated bowel from the underlying pathology.

D. If the small bowel loops fall deep into the pelvic recesses, a **PA** ⊕ **(PRONE)** film with 25 degree caudal tube angulation may be of great value. Fluoroscopy in the **PA** ⊕ **(PRONE)** position, with 15 to 20 degreees of head-down table tilt and pelvic compression, may aid spot filming of this same area.
E. If steps C and D fail to visualize these deep pelvic loops, a lateral film of the pelvis should then be used. This is reserved for last since it entails a relatively high radiation dose to the patient.

SMALL BOWEL PERFORATION

PRELIMINARY FILM: **AP ⊕ (SUPINE)** ABDOMEN

CONTRAST: 240 cc WATER SOLUBLE CONTRAST (Undiluted)

OVERHEADS: **AP ⊕ (SUPINE)** ABDOMEN

1. Place the patient in the **RIGHT LATERAL** ⊕ with the table horizontal. Have the patient start drinking or slowly administer the contrast through an indwelling NG tube. Monitor gastric distention to prevent overfilling or reflux around the NG tube.
   A. If a nasoenteric tube is already in the small bowel, start with the patient in the **AP ⊕ (SUPINE)** position and instill the contrast as fast as the small bowel motility carries it forward.

2. Obtain overhead films at 15 min. intervals (secondary to the rapid transit of water soluble contrast). Fluoroscope the abdomen at these same 15 min. intervals. Spot any areas of questionable abnormality or extravasation.

3. After the cecum is reached, take one 30 min. delayed film to R/O

delayed visualization of a small leak.

NOTES

1. If an ileocolic anastamosis is the suspected site of a leak, proceed with a water soluble enema as the first examination. This allows better distention of the anastamosis without overlapping loops obscuring the vital anatomy.

2. The role of conventional fluoroscopy in cases of suspected small bowel perforation is a very limited one. If a perforated duodenum is suspected, then the protocol for an upper GI for perforated viscus should be followed. If the suspected site of the perforation is more distal, then the examination is often less than optimal. This is because of the marked hypertonicity of the water soluble contrast that causes a fluid shift into the intestinal lumen, resulting in dilution of the administered contrast. This is in addition to the dilution caused by the normal liquid small bowel contents. Although the use of nonionic water soluble contrast theoretically would decrease the fluid shift noted above, it still cannot overcome the dilution factor of the normal small bowel contents. Therefore I think CT is of great value when a mid- to distal small bowel perforation is suspected and a diagnostic imaging study is indicated.

ILEOSTOMY STUDY

PRELIMINARY FILM: **AP ⊕ (SUPINE)** ABDOMEN

CONTRAST: LOW-DENSITY BARIUM

OVERHEADS: **AP ⊕ (SUPINE)**, STEEP **RPO** ⊗ (if ostomy is in RLQ)

EQUIPMENT: COLOSTOMY CONE WITH ATTACHED TUBING AND ENEMA BAG

1. Remove the ostomy bag. Make sure that the patient can empty, and replace this bag or have an extra one available.

2. Insert the cone and tubing as follows:
   A. Insert a lubricated, gloved finger (usually the smallest one) to determine the course of the stomal loop through the anterior abdominal wall.
   B. Extend the tubing for 5 cm past the apex of the cone.

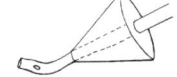

C. Gently insert the extended tubing through the stoma, aiming it in the previously determined direction until the sidehole is below the anterior abdominal wall.

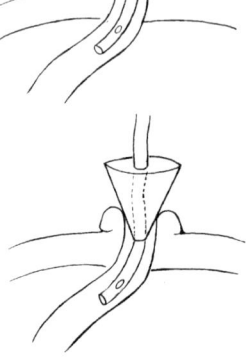

D. While holding the tubing still so that it is not pushed farther inside the patient, slide the cone down until it occludes the stomal orifice.

E. Have the patient hold the cone tightly against the stoma to prevent leakage during barium instillation and filming.

F. Slowly instill the barium with the patient in a steep **RPO** ⊘. Spot the prestomal limb of bowel in profile as it passes through the anterior abdominal wall.

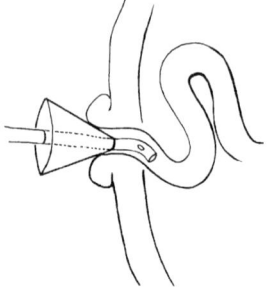

G. Continue to fill the small bowel in a retrograde manner with the patient **AP** ⊕ **(SUPINE)**.
H. Spot the right-sided loops of small bowel in a **LPO** ⊗ position and the left-sided loops in a **RPO** ⊘.

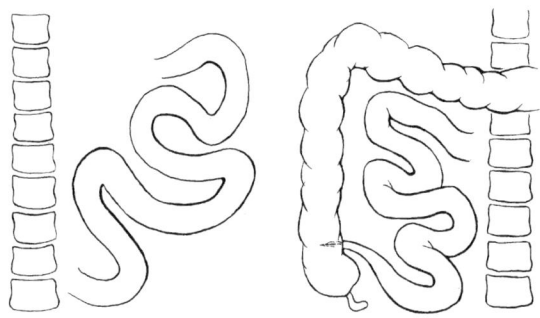

NOTES

1. Be very gentle in placing the cone and tubing. The segment of bowel that traverses the abdominal wall has limited distensibility. This is why a balloon catheter should almost never be inflated in a stomal loop.

2. The tapered conical shape of the device allows it to occlude a wide variety of stomal sizes, especially retracted ones. A prolapsed loop of bowel, posing a difficult challenge, is one of the rare indications for the use of a Foley-type catheter with an inflated balloon.

ILEOANAL "J" OR "S" POUCH

PRELIMINARY FILM: **AP ⊕ (SUPINE)** ABDOMEN

CONTRAST: WATER SOLUBLE (IF EXTRAVASATION IS SUSPECTED)

LOW-DENSITY BARIUM (IF NO EXTRAVASATION)

OVERHEADS: **AP ⊕ (SUPINE), RPO ⊗, LPO ⊗** ABDOMEN

LEFT LATERAL ⊕ RECTUM

1. Place the patient in the **LEFT LATERAL ⊕** and gently cannulate the rectum using either a small (pediatric) barium-enema tip or Foley catheter. Do not inflate the balloon on the barium-enema tip or catheter, especially if the patient is recently post-operative.

2. Slowly instill the contrast and spot the ileoanal anastamosis in the **LEFT LATERAL ⊕**.

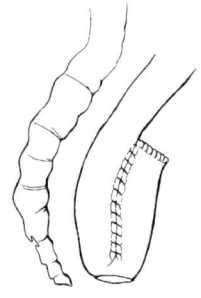

3. Turn the patient into the **LPO** ⊗ and spot the anastamosis and pouch.

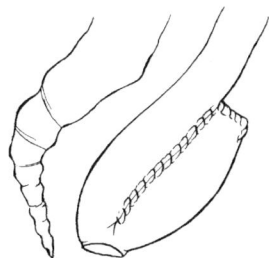

4. Place the patient in the **AP** ⊕ **(SUPINE)** and spot the anastamosis and pouch.

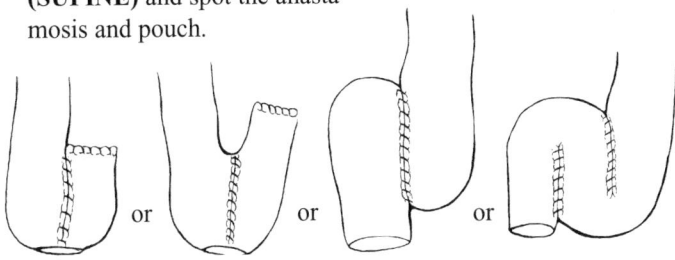

5. Continue to infuse contrast and spot some of the more proximal loops, utilizing whatever obliquity is necessary. Only fill some of these loops, since the focus of the study is usually the anastamosis and surgically created reservoir.

6. Obtain overheads.

7. If the study was performed using water soluble contrast—because of the possibility of extravasation—and none is found, then the exam of the anastamosis and pouch may be repeated with barium.

Chapter 7

COLON–ROUTINE

BARIUM ENEMA—SINGLE CONTRAST
BARIUM ENEMA—DOUBLE CONTRAST
DYNAMIC PROCTOGRAPHY (DEFECOGRAPHY)

SINGLE CONTRAST BARIUM ENEMA

PRELIMINARY FILM: **AP ⊕ (SUPINE)** ABDOMEN

CONTRAST: VERY-LOW-DENSITY BARIUM

OVERHEADS: **AP ⊕ (SUPINE), PA ⊖ (PRONE), RAO ⊗, LAO ⊗** ABDOMEN, ANGLED FILM OF THE SIGMOID, **LEFT LATERAL ⊕** RECTUM; AND **PA ⊖ (PRONE)** POST-EVACUATION.

SUBSTITUE **RPO ⊗** AND **LPO ⊗** FOR THE **RAO ⊗** AND **LAO ⊗** (if the patient cannot tolerate being turned prone)

1. Start with the table horizontal and the patient **AP ⊕ (SUPINE)**. Fill the rectum with contrast and spot.

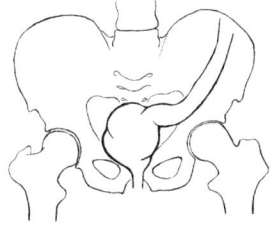

2. Turn the patient **LPO ⊗** and continue to fill the rectosigmoid and then the sigmoid. Sequentially spot the rectosigmoid junction (A), the mid-sigmoid (B), and the sigmoid-descending junction (C). Each of these spot films should in turn eliminate areas of overlapping with each curve unfurled.

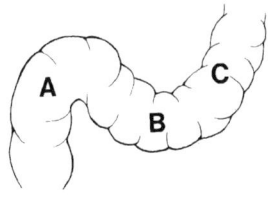

3. Turn the patient **AP** ⊕ **(SUPINE)** again and continue to fill the descending colon to a point just proximal to the radiographic splenic flexure (distal transverse colon).

4. Using fluoroscopic guidance, turn the patient **RPO** ⊘. Spot the splenic flexure with sufficient obliquity to eliminate overlapping of colonic segments along the undersurface of the flexure. This should present a smooth concavity and not an angulated appearance.

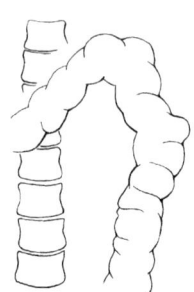

5. Return the patient to the **AP** ⊕ **(SUPINE)** position. Fill the transverse colon until the hepatic flexure is opacified and the distal ascending colon starts to fill.

6. Turn the patient **LPO** ⊘ and spot the hepatic flexure without overlapping (as in step 4).

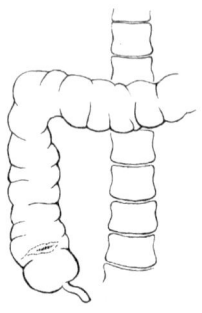

7. Turn the patient again to the **AP ⊕ (SUPINE)**. Continue to fill the ascending colon until the cecum is well-distended. The three acceptable end points of colonic filling are:
   A. Seeing the ileocecal valve.
   B. Refluxing the terminal ileum.
   C. Filling the appendix.
   Spot the cecum using external compression.

   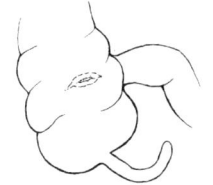

8. Using the compression paddle, compress the entire colon segmentally and sequentially. Spot any apparent fixed filling defects, irregularities, or narrowings.

NOTES

1. Use compression immediately upon seeing any defect during the filling phase of the exam. The compression paddle may be angulated to displace air bubbles or fecal material. If a defect is real, the compression adds surface detail and can help delineate a stalk or define the lesion's base.

2. During the filling phase, do not lose track of the head of the advancing barium column. This usually occurs while concentrating on obtaining spot films or trying to better distend a particular area of the colon. If a flexure or other colon segment is not fully distended during the filling phase, take a spot film. The area can be respotted after the remainder of the colon is properly filled. If one tries to fully distend the region during filling, one may lose track of the head of the column and obscure pathology such as fistularization to other segments of the GI tract.

3. As stated in *General Principles*, use glucagon to aid in filling the colon. By relieving spasm, the patient may be better able to retain the enema. It is also very helpful in differentiating spasm from a fixed narrowing.

4. The sigmoid colon may be markedly elongated and redundant. This results in multiple areas of overlapping and decreased visualization. Multiple obliquities including various degrees of **LPO** ⊗ positioning may be necessary to fully unravel these twists and turns. This is most important during fluoroscopy when small lesions can easily be overlooked or obscured by the advancing column of barium.

5. If the descending colon lies medial to the distal transverse colon at the splenic flexure, the usual **RPO** ⊘ position will actually "close" the flexure. The reverse **LPO** (⊗) obliquity will help "open" the flexure for proper spot filming.

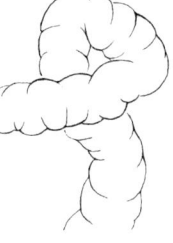

6. Due to the pressure from the overlying liver, the hepatic flexure has a more obtuse angle than the acute splenic flexure. Therefore, the degree of obliquity needed to "open" the hepatic flexure is usually much less than for the splenic flexure (which may approach the **RIGHT LATERAL** ⊕).

DOUBLE CONTRAST BARIUM ENEMA

PRELIMINARY FILM: **AP ⊕ (SUPINE)** ABDOMEN

CONTRAST: MEDIUM-DENSITY BARIUM

OVERHEADS: **AP ⊕ (SUPINE), PA ⊖ (PRONE), RIGHT LATERAL ⊕ DECUBITUS, LEFT LATERAL ⊕ DECUBITUS, UPRIGHT AP ⊕** ABDOMEN, **PRONE** CROSS-TABLE LATERAL RECTUM, ANGLED VIEW RECTOSIGMOID

1. Start with the patient in the **LAO** ⊘ position. Lower the head of the table 15 degrees. Fill the rectosigmoid colon.

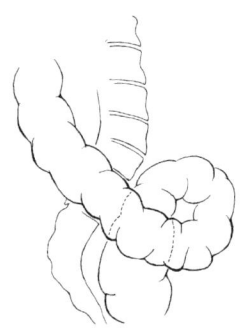

2. Continue filling the colon until the splenic flexure is reached and the barium starts to flow inferiorly and medially into the transverse colon. Stop the barium flow (see *Notes* below).

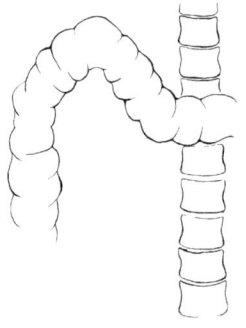

3. Turn the patient into the **LEFT LATERAL** ⊕ position. Bring the table up to the horizontal. Slowly instill the air until barium is driven into the mid-transverse colon. At this time the rectum and distal sigmoid colon should be relatively clear of barium.

4. Turn the patient into the **LPO** ⊗ position. Instill air to clear the barium from the more proximal sigmoid. Spot the air-filled rectosigmoid junction (A) and the sigmoid-descending (B) junction. Different degrees of obliquity may be needed for each area to eliminate overlapping of the adjacent segments of colon.

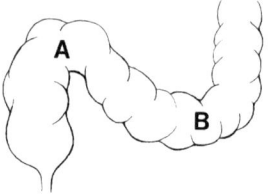

5. Turn the patient **PA** ⊕ **(PRONE)**. Continue to instill air. Check that barium fills the transverse colon to the level of the hepatic flexure. If so, then drain the barium from the rectum via siphonage (see *Notes* below). Spot the air-filled rectum in the **PA** ⊕ **(PRONE)** position.

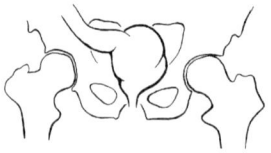

COLON—ROUTINE

6. Turn the patient into the **RAO** ⊘ position. Instill additional air and spot the air-filled rectosigmoid (A) and sigmoid-descending colon (B) junctions. As in step 4, use different degrees of the **RAO** ⊘ position to allow complete unraveling of the sigmoid turns.

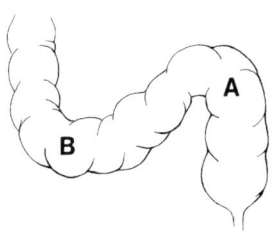

7. Turn the patient into the **RIGHT LATERAL** ⊕ position. Instill air and let the barium flow over the hepatic flexure into the ascending colon (see *Notes* below).

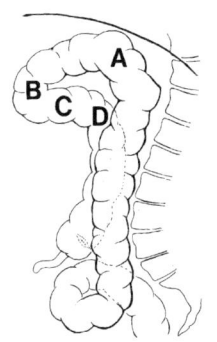

8. Turn the patient through the **RPO** ⊘ to end in the **SUPINE** (**AP** ⊕) position.

9. Elevate the head of the table 60 to 70 degrees. This allows barium to flow out of the flexures and air to rise and distend them (see *Notes* below). Turn the patient with fluoroscopic monitoring into the appropriate degree of **RPO** ⊘ that eliminates overlapping of the inferior margins of the splenic flexure. Spot the splenic flexure in this position.

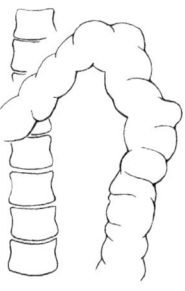

10. Return the patient to the **SUPINE (AP ⊕)** position. Locate the hepatic flexure and rotate the patient into the **LPO ⊗** position, as above. Spot the flexure without overlapping in this position.

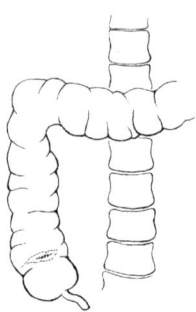

11. Return the table to the horizontal position. Spot the air-filled cecum in the **AP ⊕** or minimal **RPO ⊘**. Empty the cecum if barium-filled (see *Notes* below).

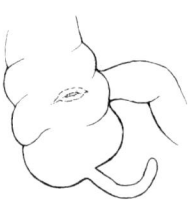

12. Turn the patient into the **LEFT LATERAL ⊕** and then **PRONE (PA ⊖)**. Drain the rectum as before and replace the air for adequate distention. Remove the rectal tube.

NOTES

1. The barium-enema tip used does not necesarily need a retention cuff attached. The retention cuff adds the potential risk—perforation of the rectum and/or damage to the anal sphincter—to an otherwise extremely safe procedure. Despite anecdotal reports to the contrary, they do not significantly increase the patient's abililty to retain the enema. The inflated retention balloon also hinders visualization of the rectal vault. This negates one of the major advantages of the double contrast enema, that of seeing the rectum in its entirety.

2. If the patient has a short sigmoid colon, then extra barium should be instilled to allow an adequate amount for filling the right colon. This usually means filling to a point between the splenic flexure and the mid-transverse colon. This holds true for both congenitally short sigmoids and post-operative colons.
   A. When the specific end point of the barium filling has been reached, the entire barium-filled column should be checked fluoroscopically. This will insure that the barium has reached the proper location without significant spasm. If spasm has forced the barium proximally, there will be insufficient contrast in the partially distended more-distal colon to properly coat the right colon. Therefore, additional barium may have to be instilled even though the barium has reached the proper level.
   B. Occasionally a redundant sigmoid colon may mimic the descending colon and the barium flow is prematurely interrupted proximal to the splenic flexure. This can be avoided by making sure that the colon along the left lateral abdominal wall is opacified to the level of the diaphragm. If this is not observed fluoroscopically in the **LAO** ⊗ projection, place the patient **PRONE (PA** ⊕ **)** and check the level of filling without the added problems of visualizing in the oblique position.

3. To drain the rectum, place the barium bag on the floor, taking care not to dislodge the rectal tube. Open the clamp on the tubing and allow the rectum to drain by siphonage. Having the patient perform a Valsalva maneuver may help. Reclamp the tubing and replace the air for adequate colonic distention. Repeat the process, if necessary. Raising the head of the table into the semi-upright position may help in the drainage. At times, the enema bag will fill with so much air that siphonage will be prevented. If this occurs, open the cap on the bag and relieve the pressure. Then resume draining.

4. At step 7, locate the air-filled splenic flexure (A) just underneath the diaphragm. With fluoroscopy follow the transverse colon inferiorly (B) along the anterior abdominal wall. It will become barium-filled as it is followed more posteriorly (C), ascending towards the hepatic flexure (D).

5. When obtaining the semi-upright spot films of the flexures, care should be taken that air-fluid levels are not present. These may obscure details in the inferior margins of the haustral sacculations. If air-fluid levels are present, the table tilt should be decreased until they disappear. The semi-upright position is a good one in which to further instill air for complete colonic distention. This is because the air flows out of the rectum and thus limits rectal distention. By decreasing the rectal distention one may control the urge to expel the contrast.

6. If the cecum is filled with too much barium to allow double contrast, it should be emptied as follows:
   A. Starting with the table horizontal, turn the patient into the **RIGHT LATERAL** ⊕ position.
   B. Lower the head of the table 15 to 20 degrees.
   C. Turn the patient **SUPINE (AP** ⊕**)** and then **LPO** ⊗.
   D. Insufflate air as you return the table to the horizontal plane.
   E. Turn the patient **SUPINE (AP** ⊕**)** or **RPO** ⊗, if necessary, and respot the cecum.

Turning the patient right-side down allows the barium to flow up the lateral wall of the ascending colon. If the patient is turned left-side down, the barium may be trapped in the cecum as it falls medially and to the left. This obviously would not accomplish the desired emptying.

DYNAMIC PROCTOGRAPHY (DEFECOGRAPHY)

PRELIMINARY FILM: NONE

CONTRAST: MEDIUM-DENSITY BARIUM PASTE
HIGH-DENSITY LIQUID BARIUM

OVERHEADS: NONE

OTHER EQUIPMENT: COMMODE WITH SPECIAL RADIOGRAPHIC FILTRATION, RAPID SEQUENCE RECORDING DEVICE, PELVIMETRY RULER, SMALL LEAD MARKER

1. The pelvimetry ruler should be placed in the longitudinal midline of the commode at a location that will allow it to be seen on the fluoroscopy screen during the exam.

2. The tubing attached to the barium paste cannister should be filled with liquid barium just prior to its insertion.

3. With the patient on a gurney in the **LEFT LATERAL** ⊕ position, slowly instill the barium liquid and paste until the entire cannister is empty or the patient cannot retain any more contrast.

4. Mark the patient's perineum with the small lead marker.

5. Rapidly transfer the patient from the gurney to the special commode. The commode should be positioned with the fluoroscopy table upright and the patient seated in the **RIGHT LATERAL** $\oplus$ position.

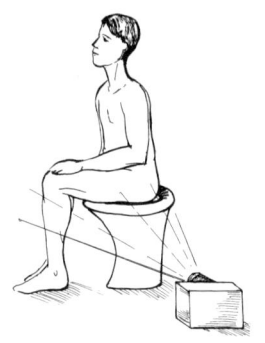

6. With the patient at rest, spot the anorectal region, making sure to include the perineal marker and pelvimetry ruler on the film.

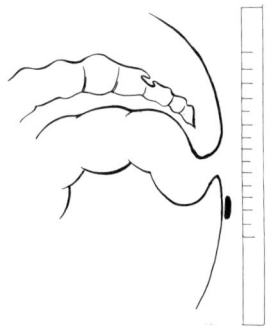

7. Have the patient "strain" by performing a Valsalva maneuver. Do not have the patient evacuate, but note any incontinence. Spot the anorectal region, as above.

8. Allow the patient to evacuate, and film this process at a rate of $1/2$ frame/sec.

9. Take a final film of the anorectal area post-evacuation, noting any residua.

10. The patient may be repositioned in the **AP** ⊕ projection and a second evacuation observed, if necessary.

NOTES

1. The special commode should be fitted with sufficient filtration so that there is rough equalization of the radiographic density of the commode and the patient's buttocks in the lateral projection. This prevents "burn-out" of the image when the area below the buttocks is included in the radiographic field.

2. The liquid barium is used to help delineate the walls of the rectum and anal canal, since the paste may occupy the middle of the lumen and not be in contact with the walls. The wall visualization is necessary to perform the various measurements of the anorectal angles and pelvic descent. The lead marker is similarly used to identify the perineum and aid in measurement of the pelvic floor descent during defecation.

3. The fluoroscopy tower must be maintained at a constant distance from both the patient and the fluoroscopy table so that the geometric magnification factor is constant as well. The sagitally-oriented pelvimetry ruler also allows exact calculation of the pelvic floor descent of the midline anorectal structures.

Chapter 8

COLON–SPECIAL

SALVAGING THE FAILED DOUBLE CONTRAST STUDY
OBSTRUCTION
PERFORATION
END COLOSTOMY
ANTERIOR RESECTION WITH RECTAL POUCH
DOUBLE-BARREL COLOSTOMY
RECTOVAGINAL FISTULA
RECTOVESICAL FISTULA
BOURNE TEST

SALVAGING THE FAILED DOUBLE CONTRAST ENEMA

The usual cause of a failed double contrast enema is insufficient and/or maldistributed barium which does not reach and coat the right colon.

1. If there is sufficient barium in the left colon but the difficulty lies in advancing it into the more proximal colon, the following procedure should be followed.
    A. Determine fluoroscopically where the largest pool of contrast is. Identify the immediate, most adjacent, and more proximal empty segment.
    B. Place that empty segment so that it is more dependent than the adjacent, filled segment. This may entail rotating the patient as well as table tilting. Allow gravity to help fill this area. If more air is needed to help propel the barium into this area, instill it slowly. If the rectum becomes overdistended with air and/or the patient has difficulty retaining the air, empty the rectum of air by venting it through the rectal tubing; and then refill gently. This cycle of air propulsion, venting, and refilling will aid

in the retrograde flow of barium. When the proximal segment is filled with contrast, and the previously filled segment is empty, reposition the patient, as above.
C. Alternate steps A and B until the cecum is reached.

2. If there is insufficient barium to coat the colon and the right colon is already distended and air-filled, follow the procedure below:
    A. Refill the enema bag with barium that has been diluted 1 : 1 with water. This can be done in the same bag originallly used, avoiding reinsertion of the enema tip.
    B. Fill the colon with the diluted barium until the proximal transverse colon is opacified.
    C. Place the patient in the **RIGHT LATERAL** ⊕ and let the ascending colon partially fill with barium.
    D. Return the patient to the **PA** ⊕ **(PRONE)** position and drain the rectum by siphonage.
    E. Perform the routine overheads for a double contrast barium enema. The addition of the diluted barium will not cause decreased coating of the colonic mucosa because it mixes with

the already instilled, nondiluted barium used in the initial attempt.

3. If there is excess fluid from the colon preparation used (especially if colonic lavage was ordered), then there is little that can be done to improve the coating. Additional turning of the patient may help a little, but it usually is insufficient to rescue the double contrast examination. At this point the examination should be converted to a single contrast study. This can be done by sending the patient to the bathroom to evacuate the medium-density barium and, more importantly, the air administered for the double contrast study. Very-low-density contrast should then be administered and a routine single contrast enema performed. It is a great disservice to continue the double contrast study and report it out as "suboptimal" and then request a repeat study or colonoscopy. Everything that can be done to improve the study should be done at the initial encounter, unless a change in the patient's condition or consent warrants a second appointment.

NOTE

1. There is no such thing as an air block. Because the colon is elastic and both elongates and distends with filling, a bubble of air cannot and does not block the flow of barium or other fluids. What actually happens is that the instilled air flows over the barium in an already partially-distended lumen without propelling the barium retrograde. To counter this phenomenon, the colon must be returned to its partially collapsed state (hence the venting described above), or the amount of fluid must be increased so that the air cannot easily flow past it. It usually takes a combination of both to overcome the problem of incomplete filling of the right colon.

COLONIC OBSTRUCTION

1. Perform the routine single contrast study (as below) with the following changes:
   A. Keep very close track of the head of the column of the advancing barium. If there is an abrupt change in the density of the barium, from its regular appearance to very dilute, check the transition point for an obstructing lesion. The dilution is probably secondary to fluid retained proximal to the level of the obstruction.
   B. If an acute angulation of the colon is seen (∗) without obvious explanation, obtain a lateral film to include the angulated area and the anterior abdominal wall. Very often these angulations are secondary to involvement in clinically occult hernias.

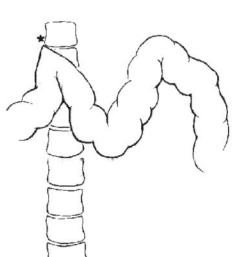
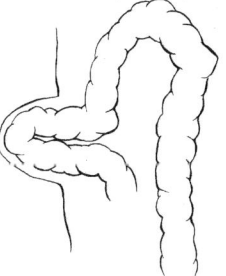

C. If an obstructing lesion is identified, do not continue to fill the colon proximal to this level. This will only result in more barium proximally, which could dessicate and impact, theoretically. In addition, the more barium retained proximal to the obstruction, the more it might interfere with the surgeon if decompression and/or resection is emergently performed.

2. Start with the table horizontal and the patient **AP** ⊕ **(SUPINE)**. Fill the rectum with contrast and spot.

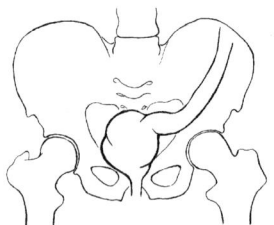

3. Turn the patient **LPO** ⊘ and continue to fill the rectosigmoid and then the sigmoid. Sequentially spot the rectosigmoid junction (A), the mid-sigmoid (B), and the sigmoid-descending junction (C). Each of these spot films should in turn eliminate areas of overlapping with each curve unfurled.

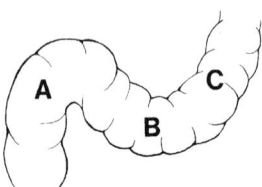

A. If the sigmoid colon enters a left inguinal hernia, there can be difficulty in filling the more proximal colon. This is the result of filling and distending the efferent limb of colon as it traverses the inguinal ring. The distended distal colon compresses the more proximal, collapsed afferent limb at this level, preventing filling. To overcome this difficulty, perform the following:

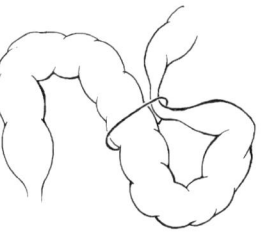

1) At the start of the procedure, manually reduce the hernia; keep the hernia reduced with manual pressure (using a lead glove for radiation protection).
2) Fill the sigmoid colon until the descending colon is reached. Remove the external compression on the hernia. Proceed as usual. Once the sigmoid colon is fully distended, it is much less likely to reenter the hernia sac.

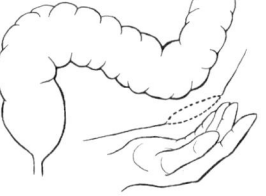

4. Turn the patient **AP ⊕ (SUPINE)** again and continue to fill the descending colon to a point just proximal to the radiographic splenic flexure (distal transverse colon).

5. Using fluoroscopic guidance turn the patient **RPO** ⊘. Spot the splenic flexure with sufficient obliquity to eliminate overlapping of colonic segments along the undersurface of the flexure. This should present a smooth concavity and not an angulated appearance.

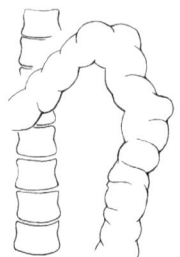

6. Return the patient to the **AP** ⊕ **(SUPINE)** position. Fill the transverse colon until the hepatic flexure is opacified and the distal ascending colon starts to fill.

7. Turn the patient **LPO** ⊘ and spot the hepatic flexure without overlapping (as in step 5).

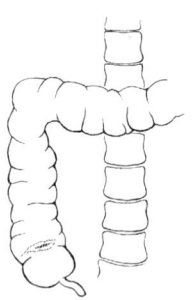

8. Turn the patient again to the **AP** ⊕ **(SUPINE)**. Continue to fill the ascending colon until the cecum is well distended. The three acceptable end points of colonic filling are:
   A. Seeing the ileocecal valve.
   B. Refluxing the terminal ileum.
   C. Filling the appendix.
   Spot the cecum using external compression.

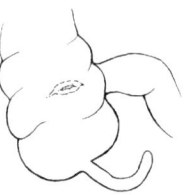

COLONIC PERFORATION

PRELIMINARY FILM: **AP ⊕ (SUPINE)** ABDOMEN

CONTRAST: WATER SOLUBLE (30% IODINATED)

OVERHEAD FILMS: **AP ⊕ (SUPINE), RPO ⊗, LPO ⊗, LEFT LATERAL ⊕ RECTUM, ANGLED VIEW** OF SIGMOID, **AP ⊕ (SUPINE)** ABDOMEN POST-EVACUATION

1. Proceed as per the routine single contrast examination, with the following caveats:
   A. Stop at the first sign of extravasation.
   B. Spot any anastamotic site, in at least two projections, as close as possible to 90 degrees apart in angulation.
   C. Do not use vigorous compression in diseased areas of the colon. Overly strong compression may actually contribute to perforation of a previously intact but compromised bowel.
   D. Examine the post-evacuation film closely for extraluminal contrast. If a leak is still suspected but not actually visualized, a 30 min. delayed film may be of value. If the kidneys are opacified on that film, it may be secondary to extravasa-

tion, absorption across the peritoneal membrane, and subsequent renal excretion. Alternatively, the contrast may be absorbed across an intact colonic mucosa entering the bloodstream in that manner.

E. If no leak is seen, even on delayed films, the entire exam may be safely repeated with barium. This may allow better visualization of diseased areas of the colon than the water soluble contrast. Barium may also allow very small fistulae or sinus tracts to be identified.

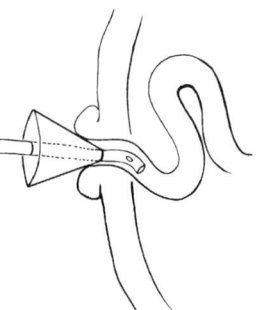

END COLOSTOMY

PRELIMINARY FILM: AP ⊕ **(SUPINE)** ABDOMEN

CONTRAST: VERY-LOW-DENSITY BARIUM

OVERHEADS: AP ⊕ **(SUPINE), RPO** ⊘, **LPO** ⊘

EQUIPMENT: COLOSTOMY CONE WITH ATTACHED TUBING AND ENEMA BAG

1. Insert the tube with the attached colostomy tip as follows:
   A. Insert a lubricated, gloved finger (usually the smallest one) to determine the course of the stomal loop through the anterior abdominal wall.
   B. Extend the tubing for 5 cm past the apex of the cone.
   C. Gently insert the extended tubing through the stoma, aiming it in the previously determined direction until the sidehole is below the anterior abdominal wall.

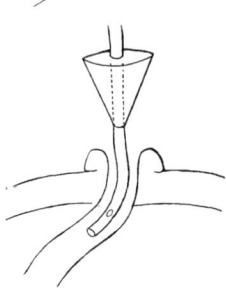

D. While holding the tubing still so that it is not pushed farther inside the patient, slide the cone down until it occludes the stomal orifice.

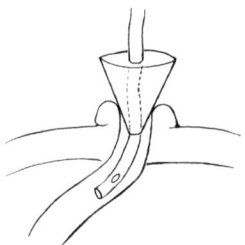

E. Have the patient hold the cone tightly against the stoma to prevent leakage during barium instillation and filming.

2. Start with the table horizontal and the patient in the **LPO** ⊗, bringing the stoma and prestomal colon into profile, perpendicular to the X-ray beam.

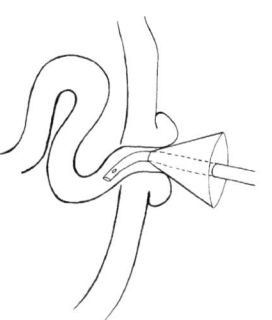

3. Start filling the prestomal loop of colon and spot its passage through the anterior abdominal wall.

4. Turn the patient **AP** ⊕ **(SUPINE)** again, and continue to fill the descending colon to a point just proximal to the radiographic splenic flexure (distal transverse colon).

5. Using fluoroscopic guidance, turn the patient **RPO** ⊗. Spot the

splenic flexure with sufficient obliquity to eliminate overlapping of colonic segments along the undersurface of the flexure. This should present a smooth concavity and not an angulated appearance.

6. Return the patient to the **AP ⊕ (SUPINE)** position. Fill the transverse colon until the hepatic flexure is opacified and the distal ascending colon starts to fill.

7. Turn the patient **LPO ⊗** and spot the hepatic flexure without overlapping (as in step 5 for the splenic flexure).

8. Turn the patient again to the **AP ⊕ (SUPINE)**. Continue to fill the ascending colon until the cecum is well distended. The three acceptable end points of colonic filling are:
   A. Seeing the ileocecal valve.
   B. Refluxing the terminal ileum.
   C. Filling the appendix.
   Spot the cecum using external compression.

9. Using the compression paddle, compress the entire colon segmentally and sequentially. Spot any apparent, fixed-filling defects, irregularities, or narrowings.

ANTERIOR RESECTION WITH RECTAL POUCH (HARTMANN PROCEDURE)

PRELIMINARY FILM: AP ⊕ **(SUPINE)** ABDOMEN

CONTRAST: WATER SOLUBLE (30% IODINATED) IF PERFORATION OR LEAKAGE IS SUSPECTED;

OR

VERY-LOW-DENSITY BARIUM

OVERHEADS: **AP ⊕ (SUPINE), RPO ⊘ , LPO ⊘**

EQUIPMENT: COLOSTOMY CONE WITH ATTACHED TUBING AND ENEMA BAG

1. The distal portion of the colon should be examined first. This is done by cannulating the rectum and proceeding cautiously with filling of the rectal stump. Start with the table horizontal and the patient in the **LEFT LATERAL** ⊕ position. Slowly fill the rectum and spot when distended. Usually the rectal pouch is small and somewhat difficult to distend fully.

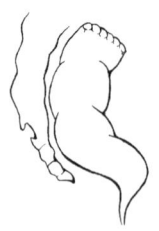

2. Turn the patient into the **AP ⊕ (SUPINE)** and spot the rectum again.

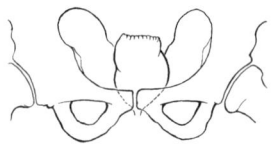

3. Drain the rectum by siphonage (placing the bag on the floor and then opening the clamp, allowing barium to flow back into the bag).

4. Cannulate the end colostomy (usually in the left mid-abdomen or lower quadrant):
   A. Insert a lubricated, gloved finger (usually the smallest one) to determine the course of the stomal loop through the anterior abdominal wall.
   B. Extend the tubing for 5 cm past the apex of the cone.

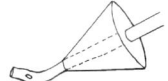

   C. Gently insert the extended tubing through the stoma, aiming it in the previously determined direction until the sidehole is below the anterior abdominal wall.

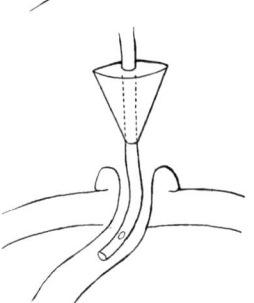

D. While holding the tubing still so that it is not pushed farther inside the patient, slide the cone down until it occludes the stomal orifice.

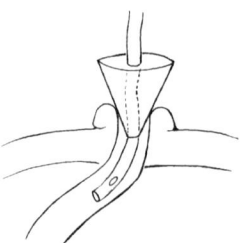

E. Have the patient hold the cone tightly against the stoma to prevent leakage during barium instillation and filming.

5. Turn the patient into the **LPO** ⊗ and slowly fill the pre-stomal segment of colon as it passes through the anterior abdominal wall. Spot this portion of colon in profile with it perpendicular to the X-ray beam.

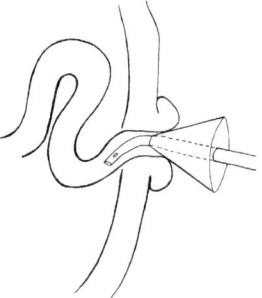

6. Turn the patient **AP** ⊕ **(SUPINE)** again and continue to fill the descending colon to a point just proximal to the radiographic splenic flexure (distal transverse colon).

7. Using fluoroscopic guidance, turn the patient **RPO** ⊘. Spot the splenic flexure with sufficient obliquity to eliminate overlapping of colonic segments along the undersurface of the flexure. This should present a smooth concavity and not an angulated appearance.

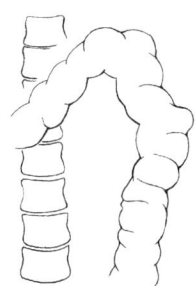

8. Return the patient to the **AP** ⊕ **(SUPINE)** position. Fill the transverse colon until the hepatic flexure is opacified and the distal ascending colon starts to fill.

9. Turn the patient **LPO** ⊘ and spot the hepatic flexure without overlapping (as in step 7 for the splenic flexure).

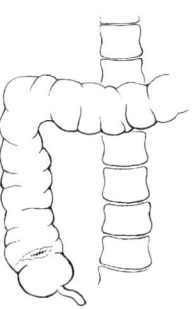

10. Turn the patient again to the **AP** ⊕ **(SUPINE)**. Continue to fill the ascending colon until the cecum is well distended. Spot the cecum using external compression.

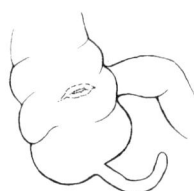

11. Using the compression paddle, compress the entire colon segmentally and sequentially. Spot any apparent fixed-filling defects, irregularities, or narrowings.

NOTES

1. If the patient is recently post-operative and a leak—especially from the rectal stump—is suspected, then water soluble contrast should be used. If the examination is a routine post-operative check, then barium should be used.
2. Keeping the rectal pouch well distended may be very difficult because of spasticity due to disuse or true diversion colitis. IV glucagon (1 to 2 mg) may be useful in decreasing the spasm.

DOUBLE-BARREL COLOSTOMY

PRELIMINARY FILM: **AP ⊕ (SUPINE)** ABDOMEN

CONTRAST: WATER SOLUBLE (30% IODINATED)
OR
VERY-LOW-DENSITY BARIUM

OVERHEADS:

A: ⊕ **(SUPINE)**, **RPO** ⊗ AND **LPO** ⊗ ABDOMEN at step 8

B: ⊕ **(SUPINE)** POST-EVACUATION FILM at step 10

C: **AP** ⊕ **(SUPINE)** and **LPO** ⊗ ABDOMEN at step 17

D: ⊕ **(SUPINE)** POST-EVACUATION FILM at step 19

EQUIPMENT: COLOSTOMY CONE WITH ATTACHED TUBING AND ENEMA BAG

1. Identify the distal limb of the colostomy, if possible. The differentiation of proximal from distal limb may be made by closely observing which limb secretes only mucus and which limb empties the fecal stream.

2. Insert the colostomy cone as follows:
    A. Insert a lubricated, gloved finger (usually the smallest one) to determine the course of the stomal loop through the anterior abdominal wall.

B. Extend the tubing for 5 cm past the apex of the cone.

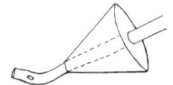

C. Gently insert the extended tubing through the stoma, aiming it in the previously determined direction until the sidehole is below the anterior abdominal wall.

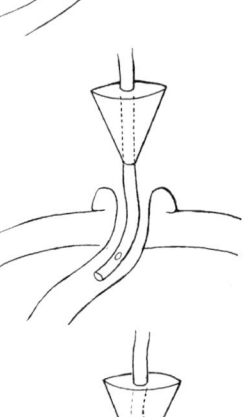

D. While holding the tubing still so that it is not pushed further inside the patient, slide the cone down until it occludes the stomal orifice.

E. Have the patient hold the cone tightly against the stoma to prevent leakage during barium instillation and filming.

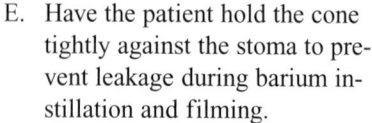

3. Turn the patient so that the stoma is seen in profile perpendicular to the X-ray beam. This most likely will be an **LPO** ⊘ if the stoma is to the left of midline; or an **RPO** ⊘, if to the right.

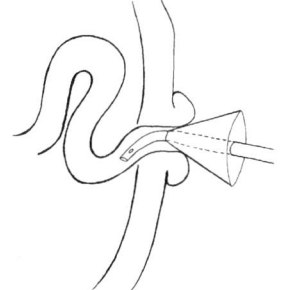

4. Slowly instill the contrast spotting the pre-stomal segment as it passes through the anterior abdominal wall.

5. Turn the patient into the **RPO** ⊘ and spot the splenic flexure, making sure that the undersurface of the flexure is a smooth concavity without overlapping of the descending and transverse colon.

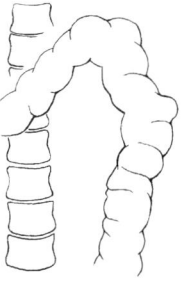

6. Return the patient to the **AP** ⊕ **(SUPINE)** position and continue to fill the colon antegrade, until the sigmoid is reached.

7. Turn the patient **LPO** ⊗ and spot the sigmoid using different degrees of obliquity to best visualize the sigmoid-descending (B) and recto-sigmoid (A) junctions. Again, these areas should be visualized without significant overlapping.

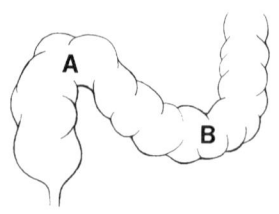

8. Overheads as above.

9. Allow the patient to evacuate the left colon by lowering the enema bag to the floor and siphoning the barium.

10. Following evacuation, obtain an overhead film.

11. Cannulate the proximal colostomy limb, using the same technique as per the ileostomy protocol.

12. Turn the patient so that the prestomal limb and stoma are viewed in profile perpendicular to the X-ray beam. Slowly fill the colon and spot the prestomal limb as it passes through the anterior abdominal wall.

13. Place the patient and fill retrograde to the hepatic flexure.

14. Turn the patient **LPO** ⊗ and spot the hepatic flexure, making sure that the undersurface is a smooth concavity without overlapping of the transverse and ascending colon.

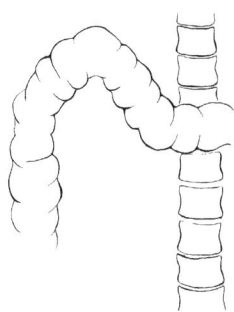

15. Return the patient to the position and continue to fill to the cecum.

16. Spot the cecum in either the **AP** ⊕ **(SUPINE)** or with minimal **LPO** ⊗ obliquity, if overlapping from the previously filled sigmoid is a problem.

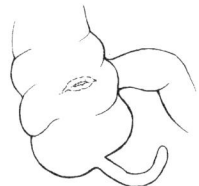

17. Obtain overheads.

18. Drain the right colon by lowering the enema bag and siphoning the barium.

19. Obtain an overhead film post-evacuation.

NOTES

1. Glucagon 1.0 mg IV may help in filling the often-spastic left colon. This spasticity is in part secondary to disuse.

2. Cannulating the distal colostomy limb first allows evaluation of the left colon without risking reflux into small bowel. The refluxed small bowel may overlap the sigmoid colon, obscuring detail.

RECTOVAGINAL FISTULA

1. Proceed with the standard single contrast barium enema protocol, with the following changes:
   A. Have the patient insert a tampon in the vagina prior to the start of the examination.

   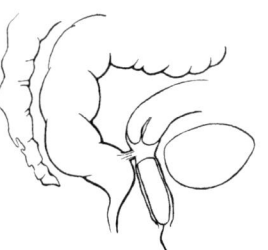

   B. Start the examination with the table horizontal and the patient in the **LEFT LATERAL** ⊕ position. Instill the barium to fill the rectum, and spot in this position.

   C. Turn the patient into the **LPO** ⊗ and fill the sigmoid colon. Continue as per the routine study.
   D. When the colon is completely filled, fluoroscope the pelvis in the **LEFT LATERAL** ⊕ position, checking for barium impregnation on the tampon.
   E. After the patient evacuates, obtain an additional post-evacuation film in the **LEFT LATERAL** ⊕ position to check for fistularization from the anterior wall of the rectum or inferior wall of the sigmoid

to the vagina without the overlapping seen in a frontal projection.

F. If there is any question of a small fistula versus an opacified loop of colon or refluxed small bowel, the tampon may be removed and a low kVp spot film of it obtained, to check for small amounts of fistularized barium.

RECTOVESICAL FISTULA

1. Proceed with the routine single or double contrast barium enema protocol, with the following changes:
   A. Start with the patient in the **LEFT LATERAL** ⊕ position and the table horizontal. Fill the rectum with barium and spot the well-distended rectum.

   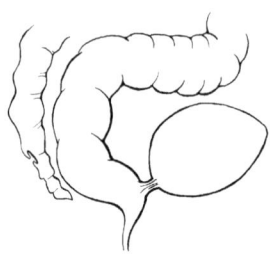

   B. Turn the patient into the **LPO** ⊗ and continue the examination as per the routine single or double contrast protocol. See the following section.

   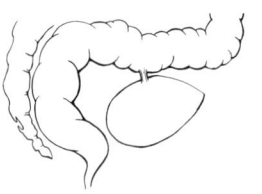

2. Perform the Bourne test if no gross filling of the bladder is appreciated under fluoroscopy. See the following section.

BOURNE TEST

The Bourne test is used as an adjunct in cases of suspected entero- or colovesical fistula.

PRELIMINARY FILMS: AS PER SBS, BE, OR ENTEROCLYSIS

CONTRAST: BARIUM AS PER SBS, ENTEROCLYSIS OR BE

OVERHEADS: **AP** ⊕ UPRIGHT OF TEST TUBES

1. After the loops of small bowel adjacent to the bladder are opacified with barium from a small bowel exam—or following patient evacuation after a barium enema—a urine sample is obtained. This may be a catheterized sample or a "clean catch" specimen without barium contamination from the perineum.

2. Centrifuge for 5 min. the urine with an identical water-filled test tube for counter-balance and comparison.

3. Take a low (approximately 60 kVp) **UPRIGHT** film of both labeled test tubes.

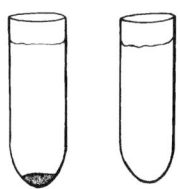

NOTE

1. If a fistula is present, the barium particles are detected in the urine sediment as radio-opaque debris at the bottom of the test tube. This technique can detect barium at dilutions of <1:100,000.

Chapter 9

PANCREAS/BILIARY TREE

ERCP
T-TUBE CHOLANGIOGRAM
NASOBILIARY TUBE STUDY
ORAL CHOLECYSTOGRAM
CHOLECYSTOSTOMY TUBE STUDY

ENDOSCOPIC RETROGRADE CHOLANGIOPANCREATOGRAPHY (ERCP)

PRELIMINARY FILM: **AP ⊕ (SUPINE)** ABDOMEN

CONTRAST: IODINATED CONTRAST (30% for CBD injections; 60% for pancreatic duct injections)

OVERHEAD: 45 MIN. DELAYED **AP ⊕ (SUPINE)** UPPER ABDOMEN

AP ⊕ (SUPINE) ABDOMEN POST-INTERVENTIONAL PROCEDURES

Preprocedure planning and cooperation with the endoscopist are vital for the successful outcome of an ERCP. Good communication is a prerequisite. Radiographic imaging should be controlled by the radiologist, who should advise the endoscopist as to the amounts of contrast and its rate of injection. The radiologist should be present for *all* injections of contrast and should be considered part of the ERCP team, not an adjunct. The endoscopist usually works with the patient in the **LAO ⊗** or **PA ⊕ (PRONE)** position (the following recommendations are based on this assumption).

CHOLANGIOGRAM PHASE

1. Use sufficient contrast to outline some intrahepatic radicles. Incomplete filling may mimic PSC, a diffuse liver process, or even cholangiocarcinoma.

2. Observe the filling of the duct during the injection of contrast. Dense contrast may flow around a defect before eventually obscuring it. Therefore, dynamic imaging may be the best clue to underlying disease.

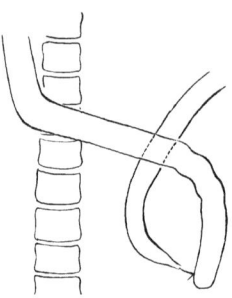

3. Small stones are best seen with dilute contrast (30 percent) and a medium kVp (~80).

4. If the endoscope obscures part of the mid-CBD, rotate the patient into a steeper **LAO** ⊘ to eliminate the overlap. If this is unsuccessful or if the patient cannot be readily moved, then have the endoscopist place a loop in the scope or straighten it to change the position or eliminate the overlapping.

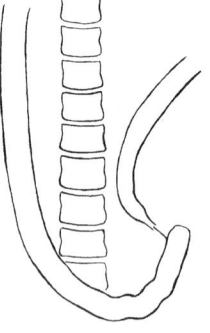

5. If the distal CBD is difficult to keep filled with contrast, despite head-down table tilt, have the patient placed SUPINE immediately following removal of the endoscope. Contrast will very often flow into the more posterior, distal CBD.

6. If a small calculus is suspected but not well seen during the initial filling phase, delayed films may show it to better advantage, since bile flow dilutes the contrast.

7. If the hepatic duct bifurcation or the right ductal system is of interest, the patient should be examined **AP ⊕ (SUPINE)** or **RPO ⊘** to allow these more-posterior ducts to fill. This will also aid in filling the distal CBD as it courses posteriorly within the head of the pancreas.

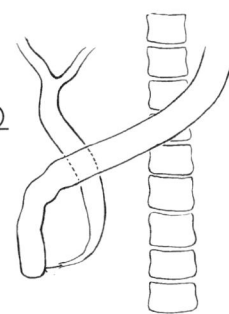

8. In the **PA ⊕ (PRONE)** or **LAO ⊘** position, the anteriorly located left ductal system is preferentially filled. If only the right system is opacified, then left ductal pathology should be suspected and further evaluated.

9. In cases of a dilated CBD or overlapping intestinal gas, external compression may be applied to allow better evaluation.

PANCREATOGRAM PHASE

1. Be alert to the possibility of a pancreas divisum so that overfilling, acinization, and the risk of pancreatitis are minimized. These may also occur in cases of ductal obstruction or inadvertant placement of the catheter in a side branch of the main duct.

2. At the junction of the main and accessory ducts, there often is an abrupt turn in the course of the duct and minimal physiologic narrowing. This may be better seen by increasing the degree of obliquity (steeper **LAO** ⊗).

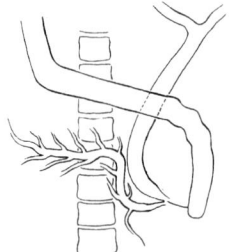

3. Along with filling of the main duct to the tail, opacification of some primary and secondary radicles is necessary to fully evaluate the organ. If the duct in the body and tail is not well-opacified and further injections of contrast not indicated or possible, turn the patient **AP** ⊕ **(SUPINE)** and the contrast will flow into those more posteriorly placed ducts.

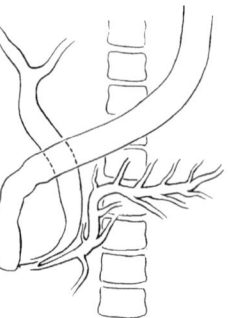

T-TUBE CHOLANGIOGRAM

PRELIMINARY FILM: **AP ⊕ (SUPINE)** OF RUQ

CONTRAST: INFUSION SETUP WITH 30% IODINE IV CONTRAST, used with medium (70–85) kVp

OVERHEADS: **AP ⊕ (SUPINE), RPO ⊘ , LPO ⊘** ALL OF THE RUQ

1. Clamp the indwelling T-tube at least 12 hr. prior to the exam.

2. With the patient **AP ⊕ (SUPINE)** on the examining table, clamp the tube 2 to 3 cm from the skin surface.

3. Cleanse the T-tube with alcohol or betadine.

4. Check the IV infusion tubing for any possible air bubbles. Purge all bubbles from the tubing. Maintain the "float chamber" at half-filled with contrast.

5. Attach a 19- to 23-gauge "butterfly" needle to the IV tubing and purge the system of bubbles again.

6. Adjust the flow through the tubing so that a slow drip from the needle tip is identified.

7. Maintaining this slow flow, place the needle into the T-tube between the skin surface and the clamp.

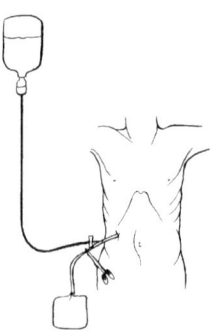

8. Shut the flow through the tubing.

9. Remove the bottle from the IV pole and lower it below table height without inverting the bottle.

10. Open the valve on the tubing slowly, aspirating bile back into the IV line. Check for air bubbles.
    A. If bubbles are seen, remove the needle from the T-tube, elevate the bottle, and start again from step 4.
    B. If no bile is aspirated, reposition the needle within the T-tube and attempt to reaspirate. If still no flow is obtained, proceed as below with a very slow infusion.

11. Replace the bottle on the IV pole and start a slow drip infusion of the contrast.

PANCREAS/BILIARY TREE 199

12. As the common bile duct (CBD) fills, and before the duodenum is opacified, spot the contrast-filled distal CBD in the **AP** ⊕ **(SUPINE)** position. Adjust the flow rate to allow adequate distention of the CBD.

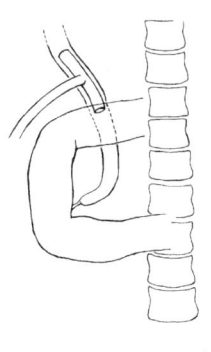

13. Turn the patient into a slight **RPO** ⊘ to prevent overlap of the distal CBD and the duodenum. Continue filling the biliary system. Spot the distal CBD as the duodenum fills.

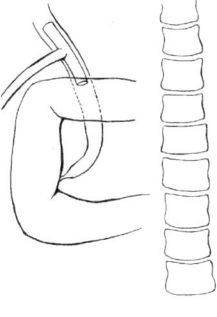

14. If the common hepatic duct and intrahepatic radicals fill, spot them in the **RPO** ⊘.

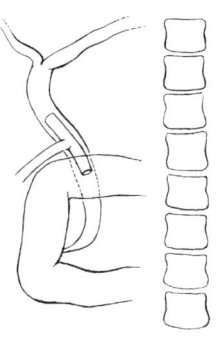

15. Spot the CHD and intrahepatic ducts in the **AP ⊕ (SUPINE)** position.

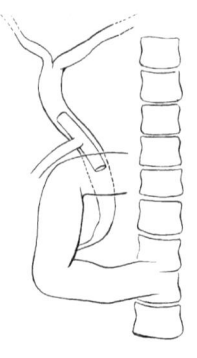

16. If the hepatic duct bifurcation is opacified, turn the patient minimally **LPO** ⊗ and respot the bifurcation and left hepatic duct. Do not rotate the patient too much, to the point that the bifurcation overlies the spine.

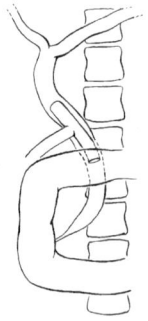

17. Slow the infusion rate, but maintain adequate ductal filling. Obtain overheads.

18. After the overhead exam is completed, stop the infusion. Lower the contrast bottle to the floor and open the valve. Allow contrast to flow retrograde in the tubing until bile is noted (ensuring adequate biliary tree decompression).

19. Shut the valve and disconnect the infusion set-up.

NOTES

1. Be aware of possible pancreatic duct filling. If this is seen, slow the infusion rate to lessen the chance of iatrogenic pancreatitis.

2. If steps 4 to 10 fail to clear the tubing of air, then air may be present in the biliary tree, either from reflux through the papilla or even the distal limb of the T-tube extending into the duodenum. Under this circumstance the best technique for a successful exam is to rapidly infuse the contrast, attempting to displace the bubbles with contrast. Both Trendelenberg and reverse Trendelenberg table-tilting may be of value.

3. DO NOT HAND INJECT CONTRAST. You can raise the intrahepatic biliary pressures excessively, causing bacteremia and possible sepsis. Gravity mediated drip infusion limits the induced hydrostatic pressures to safe levels.

NASOBILIARY CHOLANGIOGRAM

PRELIMINARY FILMS: **AP ⊕ (SUPINE), RPO ⊗** OF THE RUQ

CONTRAST: 30% IODINATED WATER SOLUBLE CONTRAST (DRIP INFUSION)

OVERHEADS: **AP ⊕ (SUPINE), RPO ⊗, LPO ⊗** OF THE RUQ

1. Run contrast through the connecting tubing from the drip infusion set-up. Purge all air bubbles from the tubing before continuing.

2. Use a 5 or 10 cc syringe to aspirate bile through the nasobiliary catheter.

3. When bile is noted at the catheter tip, insert the connecting tubing with a slow drip of contrast already running.

4. Gradually fill the biliary tree with the patient in the **RPO ⊗** position. Spot the opacified common bile duct before filling of the duodenum is obtained.

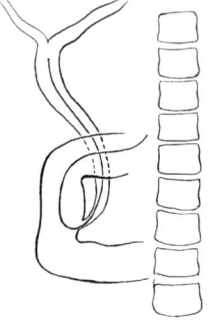

5. Continue filling the duct. If the hepatic duct bifurcation fills, spot it in the **AP ⊕ (SUPINE)** position.

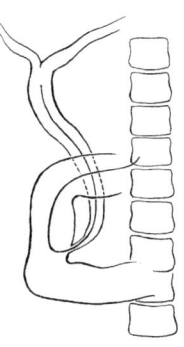

6. Turn the patient into the **LPO ⊗** and spot the left hepatic duct if it fills.

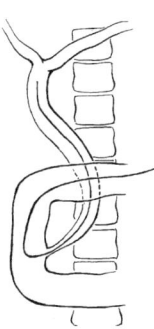

7. Obtain the overhead films.

8. Detach the connecting tubing and reconnect the drainage bag to the system.

NOTES

1. Fluoroscope and obtain both the spot films and overhead films with a kVp of approximately 70 to 75. This low kVp, combined with the medium density (30 percent iodine) contrast, allows the best visualization of small filling defects such as stones.

2. Very often aspiration is not possible due to the small diameter of the catheter and some plugging of the lumen by debris. In addition, the orifice of the tube in the biliary tree often lies against the bile duct wall and prevents aspiration.

ORAL CHOLECYSTOGRAM

PRELIMINARY FILMS: **PA** ⊕ **(PRONE)** ABDOMEN, **LAO** ⊗ OF RUQ (prior to contrast administration)

CONTRAST: ANY APPROVED ORAL CONTRAST AGENT (see *NOTES* below)

OVERHEADS: **PA** ⊕ **(PRONE)** ABDOMEN, **LAO** ⊗ OF RUQ ON DAYS 2 AND 3 (if necessary) FOR INPATIENTS; FOR OUTPATIENTS, ONLY ON DAY 3.

1. Place the table upright with the patient facing forward **(AP** ⊕**)**. Set the fluoroscopy and filming kVP at 70 to 75. Locate the contrast-filled gallbladder and spot using the compression device attached to the fluoro tower.

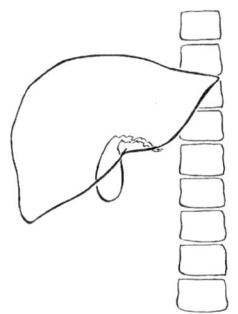

2. Take additional compression spots of the gallbladder in various degrees of **RPO** ⊗, moving it to the right of the spine and away from overlying gas.

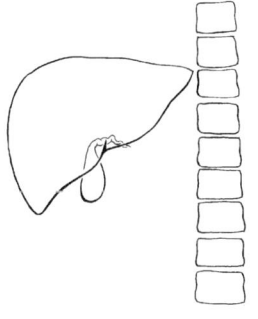

NOTES

1. If Telepaque is used as the contrast agent, then a diet including fat should be administered on the day of the tablet ingestion. No fat should then be eaten after the tablets are taken and before the filming. With other contrast agents, a fat-free diet should be followed both before and after contrast administration.

2. If gas overlies the gallbladder in all obliquities, use the compression cone in the following manner: Place the cone 5 to 8 cm below the inferior margin of the gallbladder fundus (A); compress and—while continuing the pressure—then move the cone superiorly (A′).

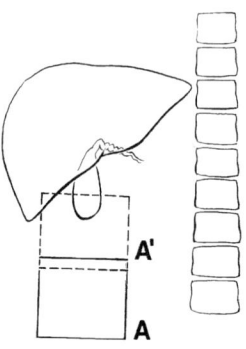

3. Outpatients are requested to come to the Radiology Department on day 3, saving them a trip on day 2, when many patients may have suboptimal visualization of the gallbladder. The preliminary films may be performed many days, or even weeks, prior to the contrast administration.

CHOLECYSTOSTOMY TUBE STUDY

PRELIMINARY FILMS: **AP** ⊕ **(SUPINE), RPO** ⊗ OF RUQ

CONTRAST: 60% IODINE DRIP FUSION CONTRAST

OVERHEADS: **AP** ⊕ **(SUPINE), RPO** ⊗ , MINIMAL **LPO** ⊗ OF RUQ

1. Determine the type of cholecystosmy tube in place.
   A. If a Foley catheter has been used, do not insert a needle into the catheter beyond the point where the balloon insufflation channel and the main catheter unite. Only use that portion adjacent to the flared end of the main lumen. If the conjoined portion is punctured, the balloon may deflate and the tube inadvertently dislodge. Proceed as per steps 3 to 11 in the T-tube cholangiogram.
   B. If a "mushroom" or straight catheter has been used, then the tip of the IV connecting tubing should gently be inserted into the open end of the catheter while a slow drip of contrast is running. This should minimize the chance of

introducing air bubbles into the tubing. Proceed as per steps 8 to 11 in the T-tube cholangiogram.

2. Start filming as per step 12 in the T-tube study.

NOTES

1. In patients with cholecystostomy tubes, there very often is gallbladder neck or cystic duct obstruction. In these patients, aspiration of bile is limited or not possible at all. If this is encountered, then proceed with a slow infusion of contrast. Check for extravasation along the catheter tract, and stop if this is seen.

2. If the above measures fail to clear the catheter and/or biliary tree of air, a rapid infusion of contrast may help purge the system and allow adequate visualization.

Chapter 10

MISCELLANEOUS

FISTULOGRAM

FISTULOGRAM

PRELIMINARY FILM: **AP ⊕ (SUPINE)** ABDOMEN

CONTRAST: 60% IODINATED CONTRAST DRIP INFUSION

OVERHEADS: **AP** ⊕, **RPO** ⊗ OR **LPO** ⊗ ABDOMEN (AS REQUIRED)

OTHER EQUIPMENT: 8 FRENCH PEDIATRIC FEEDING TUBE, VARIOUS SIZES OF FOLEY CATHETERS, SHORT ANGIOGRAPHIC 5 FRENCH CATHETERS WITH MOVEABLE CORE WIRE

1. The first principle of fistulography is that of identifying the orifice of the fistulous tract or draining sinus. Most of the time this is obvious. However, in post-operative cases with a draining wound or incision, it may be very difficult to identify what area to cannulate. When this occurs, one should "walk" the wound from one end to the other using the pediatric catheter first. Gently probe for the orifice of the underlying fistula. When an orifice is identified, slowly and gently advance the catheter through it, into its deeper recesses. If any resistance is felt, stop and hand inject a small amount of contrast to identify the problem. If the cavity is sizeable,

then the catheter may be attached to the drip infusion set-up and contrast administered.

2. Occasionally the orifice of the fistula is so large that contrast leaks out to the skin surface instead of filling the fistula or abscess cavity. In these cases a Foley catheter with an already inflated balloon may be used to administer the contrast. The balloon should be pressed against the skin surface, but not placed below it in the fistula or wound.

3. When a sizeable cavity is encountered or multiple tracts arise from a fistula or cavity, the catheter should be repositioned, exploring these areas with small test injections of contrast. These attempts may yield filling of additional unsuspected loculations or fistulae.

4. If the pediatric feeding tube is too soft to properly advance, a small-bore (5 French) angiography catheter may be substituted. A moveable core guide wire can be used judiciously with the catheter to afford the most flexibility and stability to explore a most difficult situation safely.

Appendix I

PATIENT CHECKLIST

*Patient Name*_____
*Unit#*_____ *Resident*_____

	YES	NO
1. If female and childbearing age, is patient pregnant?		
2. Difficulty in swallowing? If yes, solids? If yes, liquids? At what level?_____		
3. Is there abdominal pain? If yes, where? If yes, when?		
4. Does patient have nausea/vomiting? If yes, is there blood, coffee grounds?		
5. Is there recent change in bowel habits? If so, diarrhea? If so, constipation?		
6. Is there melena or BRBPR?		

	YES	NO
7. Has there been recent change in weight? If so, intentional? If not, ? lbs. _____ In ? wks. _____		
8. What medications/drugs does patient take?		
9. Does patient have any allergies? If so, to what?		
10. Does patient drink EtOH? If so, how much?		
11. Does patient smoke? If yes, how many pack/day?		

12. Has patient had prior surgery?
If yes, Appendectomy?
    Cholecystectomy?
    Billroth II?
    Colon resection?
    Other?_____		

FLUOROSCOPIC FINDINGS

SMALL BOWEL SCHEDULE (fill in actual time obtained)

Immediate_____ 15 min._____ 30 min._____
60 min._____ 90 min._____ 120 min._____
180 min._____ Others_____

Appendix II

SAMPLE REPORT

PATIENT DEMOGRAPHICS

History: 37-year-old male with acute onset mid-epigastric pain and GI bleeding.

Report: Preliminary film of the abdomen was unremarkable.

Following the IV administration of 0.1 mg. of glucagon, the patient ingested gas-forming granules and barium for a double contrast upper GI series.

Barium passed through the esophagus without delay or obstruction. No constant filling defect or irregularity of the esophagus was noted. No hiatal hernia or significant gastroesophageal reflux was seen.

The stomach was normal in position and showed good peristalsis. A large (3.5×4.1 cm), irregular intraluminal mass was noted along the lesser curvature of the distal antrum. The mass made acute angles with the remainder of the stomach and extended through the pylorus to involve the base of the duodenal bulb. An irregular, eccentric collection of barium was seen within this mass. The apex of the duodenal bulb and the sweep were unremarkable.

>The findings in the stomach suggest a primary malignancy. Although lymphoma crosses the pylorus more frequently than adenocarcinoma, the greater prevalence of the latter makes it the more likely diagnosis.

Conclusion: Malignant neoplasm of the distal antrum and bulb, most likely adenocarcinoma.

REPORT GUIDLINES

1. The report is divided into four distinct parts. The first is *Demographics*, including the patient's name, medical record number, sex, date of birth, etc. The exact order and type of data presented vary from institution to institution and very often are downloaded from either an RIS (Radiology Information System) or an HIS (Hospital Information System).

2. The second portion is that of appropriate clinical information, here entitled *History*. In many institutions and practices, this is also downloaded via electronic means; in others, it may be part of the request for the examination. In yet other practices, it may have to be entered by the radiologist as part of the dictation. Because most radiologists do not maintain separate and distinct office notes in their practice, this section may be the only record of why the procedure was being done, and what clinical information was available to the radiologist at the time of interpretation. This may be very important information to have in a contemporaneous record in our litigious society.

3. The *Report* has many subdivisions. If a preliminary film was obtained, it should be reported as part of the complete examination. The reporting radiologist is responsible for all pertinent information contained on that film.

   Any medication that was given to the patient should be reported as to the name of the drug, its dosage, and route of administration. Any side effects should be reported in this section. If the patient's chart is available, a progress note documenting this administration should also be written.

The next portion of this section should contain a description of the radiographic findings. This should include pertinent negatives, tailored to the appropriate clinical situation. The analysis follows the descriptive portion of the report. The radiologist should discuss the reasons why a certain diagnosis is favored, and what, if any, differential diagnoses should also be considered.

4. Although there is some disagreement as to what is the proper terminology for the concluding portion of a radiology report, I believe that *Conclusion* is as appropriate as any alternative. This final part ends the report, usually conveying in a short declaration a summary of the radiologist's findings.

5. The question of whether or not the radiologist should make recommendations within the report, as to further testing or therapy, is subject to much heated debate. I prefer to make my concerns known in writing, directly to the referring physician. Many non-radiologists feel that their "hands are tied" once a recommendation is made in print. In other cases, some radiologists would argue that a problem case is best discussed frankly and completely without a written record being made.

This very often contradicts the advice of legal counsel and risk managers. In addition, this entire topic is subject to reinterpretation in light of the new ACR guidelines for reporting of mammography results, in which the radiologist is considered an active participant in recommending follow-up procedures, whether imaging-related or not.

Appendix III

PATIENT POSITIONING GUIDE

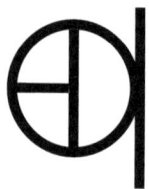

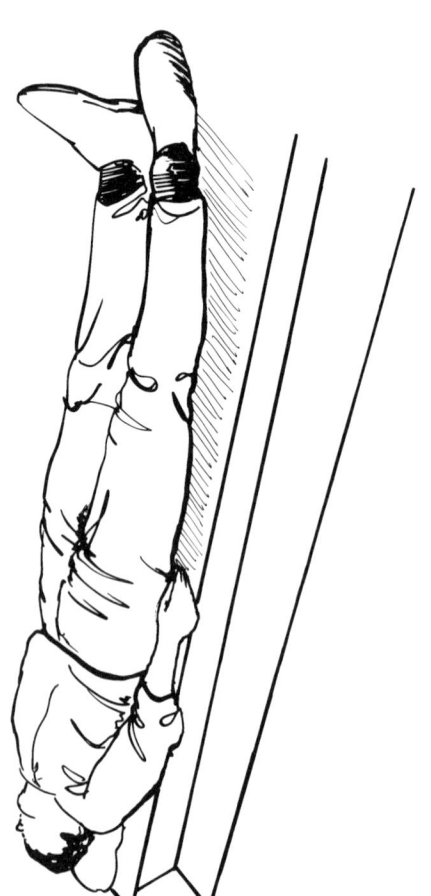

AP SUPINE

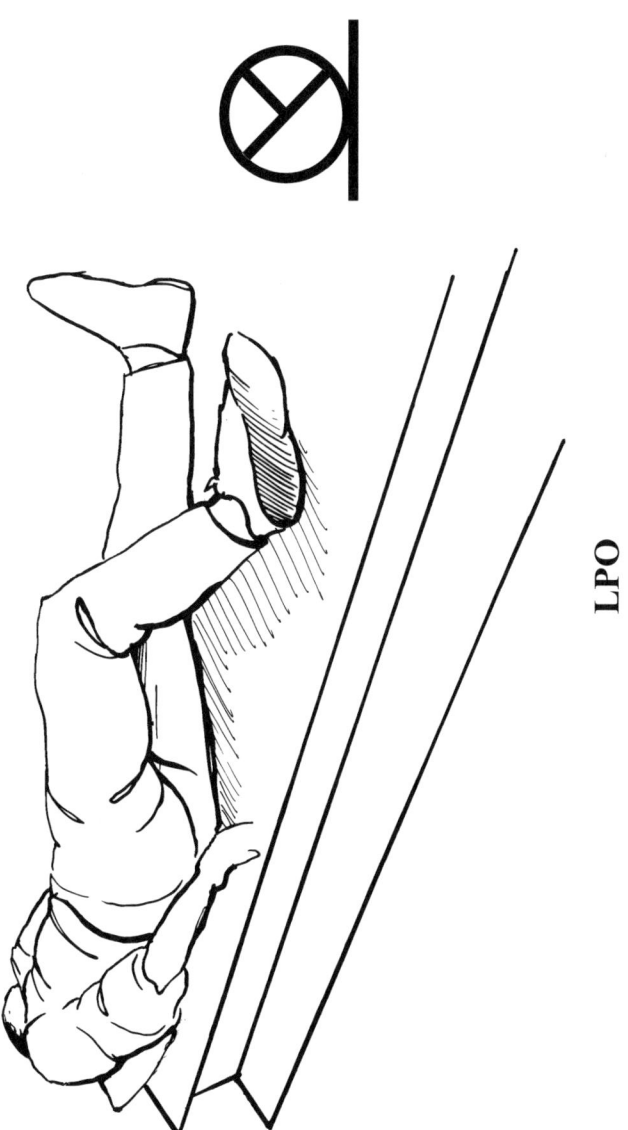

LPO

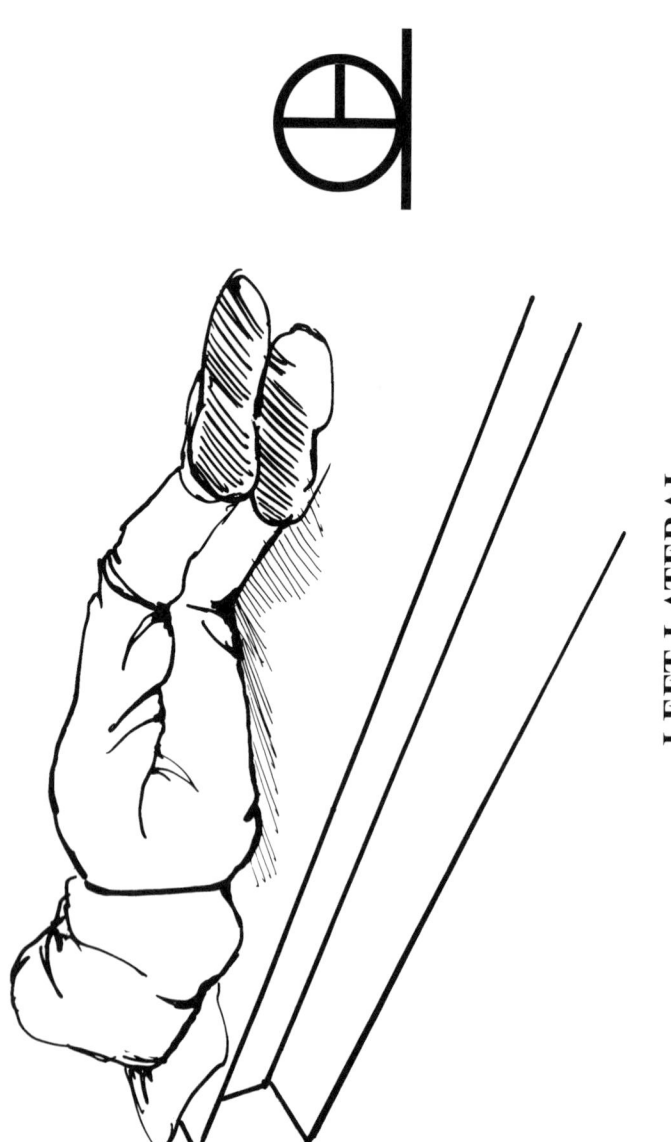

LEFT LATERAL

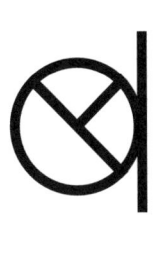

LAO

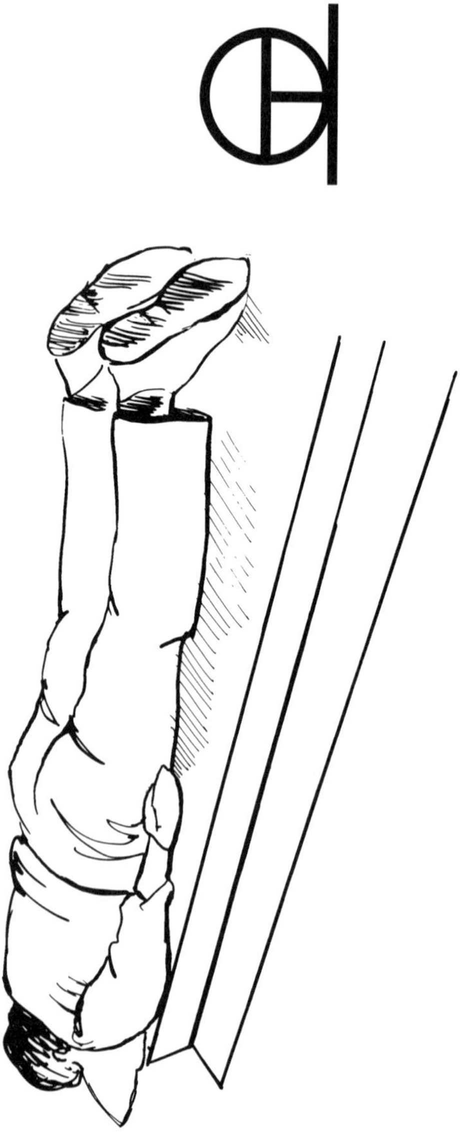

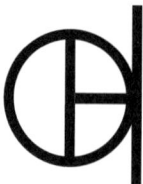

PA

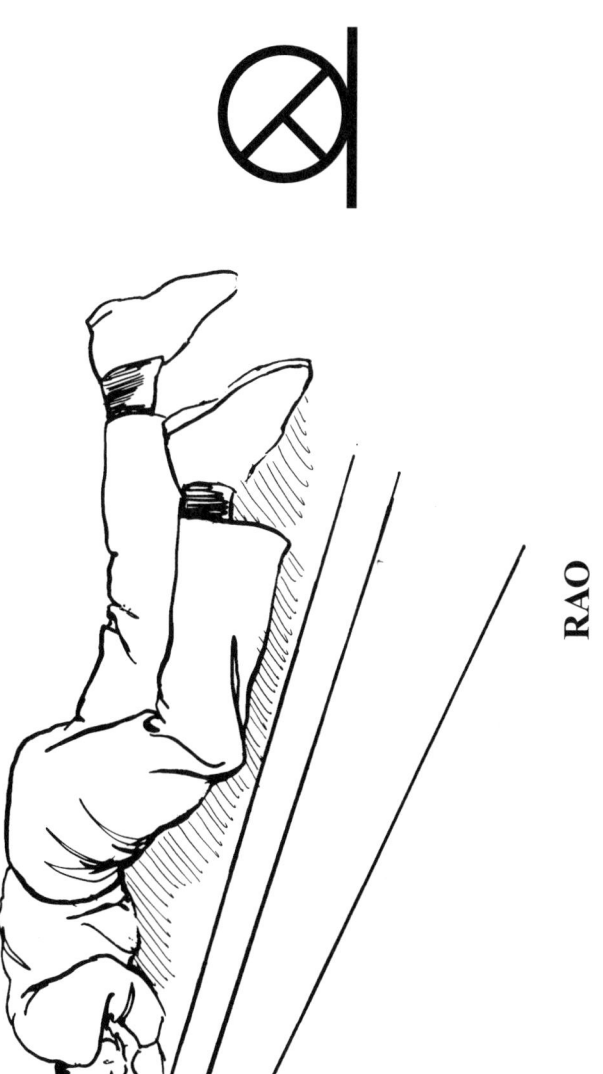

RAO

RIGHT LATERAL

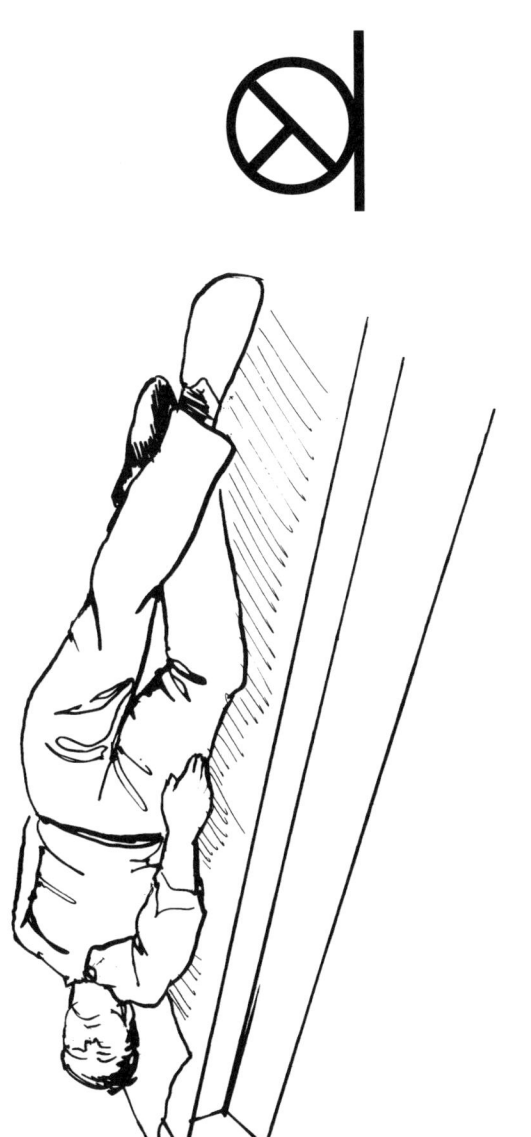

RPO

INDEX

A
Achalasia, 38

B
Barium:
   densities, 19
   penetration of by X-ray, 4
   percent w/v in Japan, 6, 7
   types of, 19
Barium enema:
   and post-evacuation film, 16
   double contrast, 151
   failed, salvaging the, 163
   preparation, 13
   single contrast, 147
Biliary tree/pancreas, 191–208:
   cholangiogram, nasobiliary, 202; t-tube, 197
   cholangiopancreatography, endoscopic retrograde (ERCP), 193
   cholecystogram, oral, 205
   cholecystostomy tube study, 207
Billroth II:
   double contrast, 93
   single contrast, 90

Bowel, small:
   enteroclysis, 117, 124, 127
   ileoanal "J" or "S" pouch, 142
   ileostomy study, 139
   obstruction, 135
   perforation, 137
   routine, 111–130
   special, 131–143
   study, dedicated, 113
   tube placement, enteroclysis, 117
Bourne test, 189
Bulb, posterior duodenal, maneuver, 83

C
Celestine tube implant study, 58
Cholangiogram:
   nasobiliary, 202
   t-tube, 197
Cholangiopancreatography, 193
Cholecystogram, oral, 205
Cholecystostomy tube study, 207
Colon:
   barium enema, 147, 151
   interposition, post-colonic, 56

Colon: *(continued)*
  obstruction, 167
  perforation, 171
  routine, 145–159
  special, 161–190
Colostomy:
  double-barrel, 181
  end, 173
Compression, contraindications to, 14
Contrast studies:
  comparison, single vs. double, 5, 8
  comparison, water soluble vs. barium, 10
  double, 5
  single, 4
  water soluble, 10

D

Defecography (proctography), dynamic, 157
Double vs. single contrast, 5,8
Duodenal bulb, posterior, maneuver, 83

E

Enema:
  agents compared, 13, 35
  failed, salvaging the, 163
Enteroclysis:
  double contrast, 127
  single contrast, 124
  tube placement, 117
Esophagogastrectomy, post-, 46
Esophagojejunostomy, post-, 52
Esophagram, cervical, rapid sequence, 25

Esophagus:
  cervical, 25
  double contrast, 30
  fistula, tracheoesophageal, 44
  foreign body, retained, 41
  obstruction, 35
  perforation, 36
  single contrast, 28
  varices, 40
Esophagus and pharynx:
  routine, 21–30
  special, 33–60

F

Films:
  spot, and overheads, 17
  post-evacuation, 16
Fistula:
  colo- or enterovesical. *See* Bourne test.
  rectovaginal, 186
  rectovesical, 188
  tracheoesophageal, 44
Fluoroscopy units, 7
Foreign body, esophageal, retained, 41

G

Gastrointestinal (GI) series, upper:
  double contrast, 68
  duodenal bulb, posterior, maneuver, 83
  perforated viscus, 88
  salvaging failed double contrast, 79
  single contrast, 63

stapling, gastric, 109
Gastrojejunostomy without resection:
bypass, 100
double contrast, 104
Gastrostomy tube, 98
Glucagon, how to use, 12

H

Hartmann procedure, 176

I

Ileoanal "J" or "S" pouch, 142
Ileostomy study, 139
Interposition, post-colonic, 56

J

"J" or "S" pouch, ileoanal, 142

N

Nasobiliary cholangiogram, 202

O

Obstruction:
colonic, 167
esophageal, 35
outlet, 86
small bowel, 135
See also Achalasia; Foreign body.

P

Pancreas/biliary tree, 191–208:
cholangiogram, nasobiliary, 202
cholangiogram, t-tube, 197
cholangiopancreatography, endoscopic retrograde (ERCP), 193
cholecystogram, oral, 205
cholecystostomy tube study, 207
Patients:
biopsied, recent, 18
females, childbearing, 11
heart disease, 18
HIV positive, 19
Perforated viscus, 88
Perforation:
colonic, 171
esophageal, 36
small bowel, 137
Pharyngogram, 23
Pharynx and esophagus:
routine, 21–30
special, 33–60
Pneumocolon, peroral, 133
Positioning patients, 19.
See also Appendix III.
Post-esophagogastrectomy, 46
Post-esophagojejunostomy, 52
Preliminary (scout) films, 1
Proctography, dynamic (defecography), 157

R

Radiation dose:
examiner, minimizing, 3
females, childbearing, 11
Reports, of examinations, 17
Resection, anterior, with rectal pouch, 176

S

"S" or "J" pouch, ileoanal, 142
Scout films. See Preliminary films.

Single vs. double contrast, 5, 8
Small bowel. *See* Bowel
Solid column studies. *See* Contrast studies, single.
Stapling, gastric, 109
Stomach:
    Billroth II, 90, 93
    duodenal bulb, posterior, maneuver, 83
    gastrointestinal (GI) series, upper, 63, 68
    gastrojejunostomy without resection, 100, 104
    gastrostomy tube, 98
    obstruction, outlet, 86
    routine, 61–75
    special, 77–109
    stapling, gastric, 109
    viscus, perforated, 88

T

Tracheoesophageal fistula, 44

Tube:
    cholecystostomy, study, 207
    enteroclysis, placement, 117
    gastrostomy, 98
    nasobiliary, 202
    t-tube, 197

U

Upper GI series:
    double contrast, 68
    duodenal bulb, posterior, maneuver, 83
    perforated viscus, 88
    salvaging failed double contrast, 79
    single contrast, 63

V

Varices, esophageal, 40
Viscus, perforated, 88